Collaborative Community Approaches to Addressing Serious Violence

Collaborative Community Approaches to Addressing Serious Violence

Editors

Jaimee Mallion
Erika Gebo

MDPI • Basel • Beijing • Wuhan • Barcelona • Belgrade • Manchester • Tokyo • Cluj • Tianjin

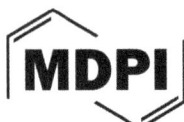

Editors

Jaimee Mallion
London South Bank University
UK

Erika Gebo
Suffolk University
USA

Editorial Office
MDPI
St. Alban-Anlage 66
4052 Basel, Switzerland

This is a reprint of articles from the Special Issue published online in the open access journal *Societies* (ISSN 2075-4698) (available at: https://www.mdpi.com/journal/societies/special_issues/ Collaborative_Community).

For citation purposes, cite each article independently as indicated on the article page online and as indicated below:

LastName, A.A.; LastName, B.B.; LastName, C.C. Article Title. *Journal Name* **Year**, *Volume Number*, Page Range.

ISBN 978-3-0365-6221-6 (Hbk)
ISBN 978-3-0365-6222-3 (PDF)

Contents

About the Editors

Jaimee Mallion

Jaimee Mallion specializes in developing prevention and intervention strategies for gang members. She focuses on strengths-based approaches to offender intervention, including the application of the Good Lives Model. This model suggests all individuals have life priorities, and when these cannot be achieved prosocially, they instead pursue these through offending behaviors. Supporting the attainment of these life priorities through prosocial means will reduce offending. Jaimee emphasizes the need for a collaborative, multidisciplinary approach within communities to support the prevention of offending.

Erika Gebo

Erika Gebo believes in active scholarly engagement with the wider community. She does so by conducting funded multidisciplinary grant work on issues related to youth justice and assistance for communities responding to violence. Her current research is conducted in collaboration with communities engaged in preventing violence. She also is interested in how institutions, such as schools and community agencies, can inhibit or promote healthy behaviors. The implications for practice and policy are important lines of research.

Preface to "Collaborative Community Approaches to Addressing Serious Violence"

As a pervasive social problem affecting communities worldwide, violence has been classified as a leading international public health problem, which requires immediate intervention (World Health Organization, 2002). By bringing together partners with varied skills, whole-system multiagency approaches are advocated as the leading means of targeting serious violence. This special issue considers the need for a collaborative approach to violence intervention within communities, focusing on domestic, sexual and youth violence. The contributions describe community-level collaborative approaches to preventing and reducing serious violence. Successes and lessons learned from the approaches are identified, and the transportability of the approaches to other locations are explored. Contributions are written by both researchers and clinicians specializing in community interventions targeting violence. It will be of interest to anyone working with perpetrators or victims of violence, as well as those researching gang, domestic or sexual violence. We want to thank all of the authors for their important contributions to this special issue, each of which demonstrate the need for a collaborative approach to addressing serious violence in the community.

Jaimee Mallion and Erika Gebo
Editors

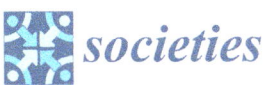

Concept Paper

Good Lives Model: Importance of Interagency Collaboration in Preventing Violent Recidivism

Jaimee Sheila Mallion

Division of Psychology, School of Applied Sciences, London South Bank University, London SE1 0AA, UK;
mallionj@lsbu.ac.uk

Abstract: Violence is a complex and multifaceted problem requiring a holistic and individualized response. The Good Lives Model (GLM) suggests violence occurs when an individual experiences internal and external obstacles in the pursuit of universal human needs (termed primary goods). With a twin focus, GLM-consistent interventions aim to promote attainment of primary goods, whilst simultaneously reducing risk of reoffending. This is achieved by improving an individuals' internal (i.e., skills and abilities) and external capacities (i.e., opportunities, environments, and resources). This paper proposes that collaborations between different agencies (e.g., psychological services, criminal justice systems, social services, education, community organizations, and healthcare) can support the attainment of primary goods through the provision of specialized skills and resources. Recommendations for ensuring interagency collaborations are effective are outlined, including embedding a project lead, regular interagency meetings and training, establishing information sharing procedures, and defining the role each agency plays in client care.

Keywords: good lives model; violence; intervention; interagency collaboration

Citation: Mallion, J.S. Good Lives Model: Importance of Interagency Collaboration in Preventing Violent Recidivism. *Societies* **2021**, *11*, 96. https://doi.org/10.3390/soc11030096

Academic Editor: Gregor Wolbring

Received: 25 June 2021
Accepted: 9 August 2021
Published: 11 August 2021

Publisher's Note: MDPI stays neutral with regard to jurisdictional claims in published maps and institutional affiliations.

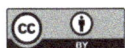
1. Introduction

Violence is a pervasive problem affecting all communities world-wide, with nearly half a million people losing their lives to intentional homicide annually [1]. Critically, this figure is on the rise: between 2015 and 2017, a four percent increase in homicide rates was recorded globally [2]. However, intentional homicide is only one form of interpersonal violence. As defined by the World Health Organization [3], violence is "the intentional use of physical force or power, threatened or actual, against oneself, another person, or against a group or community, that either results in or has a high likelihood of resulting in injury, death, psychological harm, maldevelopment or deprivation". Thus, violence incorporates acts of physical, sexual, and/or psychological abuse [4], of which homicide is not often the primary outcome.

Violence has a long-term impact on the lives of many individuals. For instance, one third of women have experienced violence from an intimate partner (IPV) during their lifetime [5], whilst approximately one billion children (aged 2–17 years) have experienced abuse in the past year [6]. In addition to the risk of serious physical harm, these acts of violence are associated with a variety of poor outcomes for the victims, including high rates of depression, anxiety, PTSD, substance misuse, and suicidality [7]. Furthermore, individuals exposed to violence are more likely to have difficulty securing and maintaining employment and be at risk of poor health outcomes later in life (i.e., health conditions related to poor coping strategies and health risk behaviors, such as diabetes, strokes, and heart attacks [8]). This highlights that the consequences of violence are long reaching, continuing to affect victims throughout their lifetime.

In addition to the direct impact on the victim, the outcomes of violence are wide reaching, deeply impacting families, friends, and communities [4]. For instance, youth violence has been well-recognized for its impact on the wider community. In areas with high rates of youth violence, community members report decreased feelings of safety, normalization of violence, and increased community stigmatization which, in turn, reduce education and employment opportunities [9]. Critically, this leads to a cyclic pattern of violent behavior, whereby younger members of the community perceive violence as an acceptable and readily available option [10,11]. Those that engage in youth violence are also more likely to perpetrate IPV and child maltreatment than their non-violent counterparts [12,13].

Previously, the pervasiveness of violence led to the perception that it was inevitable within human society, with it falling on law enforcement to respond to violent acts after the fact [4]. However, there has been a growing body of research surrounding the underlying causes of violent behavior. Taking a multifaceted approach, violence occurs from the interplay between the individual, family, peers, education, and community. Regarding the individual, factors such as impulsivity, poor emotion recognition, and substance misuse increase the risk of engaging in violence [14]. Familial incarceration, child maltreatment, and witnessing IPV are predictive factors of engaging in violent behavior [15–17]. Similarly, peer engagement in gangs, bullying, and peer substance misuse are risk factors for violence [18–20]. Regarding the education domain, poor relationships with teachers, suspension/exclusion from school, and a lack of academic attainment are associated with violent behavior [21–23]. Finally, residing in communities with high rates of violence, presence of gangs, and crime increase the risk of engaging in violent behavior [24].

As violence is a complex and multifaceted problem, there is no single solution for this issue. For too long, the response to violence (and its risk factors) has been fragmented [4]. To tackle violence, a 'whole-systems' approach is needed, whereby the various determinants (individual, family, education, peer, and community) are all examined and targeted. To enable this, a collaborative approach is necessary as various organizations have different skills, abilities, and resources, meaning they are more suited to support specific needs of an individual displaying violent behavior. For instance, social services (also known as child welfare agencies) would be best placed to provide family-based interventions, whilst educational services can advance an individual's training needs and improve access to employment. By pulling together these different organizations, this will enhance the effectiveness of violence prevention and intervention programs [25].

The aim of this paper is to emphasize the need for collaborative approaches to prevent and reduce violent behavior. To explore the benefits of interagency collaboration, it is first necessary to understand what factors can lead to engagement in violent behavior. The Good Lives Model (GLM) is one approach that can be used to understand this [26]. Unlike fragmented approaches to violence intervention, the GLM takes a holistic approach, viewing individuals as having a variety of needs/goals they are working towards attaining. When something goes wrong in the pursuit of these needs/goals, offending behavior (including violence) can occur [27]. As such, the GLM suggests that supporting individuals to attain primary goods through prosocial means will reduce the need to engage in violent behavior.

Critically, individuals present a variety of needs and goals, as well as obstacles preventing the prosocial attainment of these. Targeting all of these in an intervention can be beyond the scope of a single agency. As such, the current paper supports the assumption that interagency collaboration (i.e., collaboration between psychological services, criminal justice systems, social services, education, community organizations, and healthcare), when done well can enhance the effectiveness of violence interventions by improving access to specialized skills and resources [28]. This paper will first explain the assumptions of the GLM in relation to violent behavior. Second, the formulation and effectiveness of GLM-consistent interventions for violent behavior will be summarized. Third, research surrounding the effectiveness of interagency collaborations in offender interventions will be discussed. Finally, the implementation of interagency collaborations in GLM-consistent interventions for violent behavior will be considered, with recommendations made to carry this out effectively.

2. Good Lives Model: An Overview of Assumptions

Devised as a strengths-based framework for offending behavior interventions, the GLM proposes that the risk of offending lessens when an individual has a sufficient level of capabilities and strengths to achieve their personal goals and needs [26,29]. According to the GLM, healthy human functioning is conceptualized as the pursuit of specific goals and needs (termed primary goods), which are fundamental for survival, establishing social networks, and reproducing [30]. These primary goods are prudential in nature; rather than inherently moral goods, primary goods are experiences, characteristics, and mental states that enable an individual to have a sense of fulfilment, well-being, and happiness [31]. Based on the literature surrounding human needs [32], 11 primary goods have been identified to date (see Table 1). These primary goods are multi-faceted, meaning each of the 11 primary goods resembles a cluster of smaller components (e.g., the primary good of Relatedness includes sub-goods of having a sense of love, intimacy, emotional connection, and friendship [27]).

Table 1. Definitions of 11 Primary Goods, according to the GLM.

	Primary Good	Definition
1	Life	Basic needs for survival, physical well-being, and functioning.
2	Knowledge	Feeling well informed about matters important to the individual.
3	Excellence in Work	Pursuing personally meaningful work that enables a sense of mastery.
4	Excellence in Play	Pursuing recreational activities which gives a sense of enjoyment and skill development.
5	Excellence in Agency	Establishing a sense of autonomy, power, and independence.
6	Community	Having a sense of belonging with a wider social network, who have similar interests and values.
7	Relatedness	Connecting with others in a warm and affectionate manner (including intimate, romantic, and family relationships and friendships).
8	Inner Peace	Feeling free from emotional turmoil and stress, and effectively managing negative emotions
9	Pleasure	Sense of happiness and contentment in one's current life.
10	Creativity	Expressing oneself through novel and creative means.
11	Spirituality	Finding a sense of meaning and purpose in life.

Secondary goods (also known as instrumental goods) represent the ways in which individuals achieve their primary goods. For example, the primary good of Community could be secured by joining a neighborhood-led group (e.g., Scouts). However, the GLM suggests offending behaviors occur when primary goods cannot be adequately secured through prosocial means. This is due to weaknesses within the individual and/or their environment preventing them from achieving primary goods through appropriate methods, meaning inappropriate means are instead utilized [26]. For instance, an individual could attempt to gain a sense of Community by engaging in offending behaviors such as joining a street gang [33], which give individuals a sense of control over and status within their neighborhood, whilst simultaneously allowing them to create strong emotional connections with peers [34]. Similarly, sharing of violent and sexualized images online fosters feelings of belonging, enabling a sense of Community, as individuals connect with other like-minded people who share and validate their antisocial attitudes and beliefs [35].

Two routes leading to the use of offending behavior as a means of securing primary goods have been proposed [36]. Firstly, the direct pathway suggests offending behavior is actively utilized to attain primary goods. For example, an individual who lacks the capabilities to maintain healthy relationships may purposefully engage in violent and/or controlling behavior to prevent the relationship ending. Comparatively, according to the indirect pathway, in the pursuit of primary goods something goes awry which causes a cascading effect, resulting in offending behavior. For instance, if, when attempting to fulfil the primary good of Relatedness, an individual experiences peer rejection from prosocial groups, they may utilize maladaptive coping strategies (e.g., consumption of alcohol and drugs and/or associating with delinquent peers). The use of these maladaptive coping strategies then increases the likelihood of engaging in violent behavior [37]. Whilst violence can result from both the direct and indirect pathway, individuals' whose behavior was a product of the indirect pathway struggle most in understanding the causes of their offending behavior and may require more support to prevent recidivism [38].

To date, there have been four obstacles identified which can lead to difficulty fully attaining primary goods in a prosocial manner: use of inappropriate means, and a lack of scope, coherence, and/or capacity [39]. As highlighted above, when prosocial opportunities seem inaccessible, inappropriate means may be used in an attempt to attain primary goods. However, when antisocial secondary goods are used, the primary good is not fully secured, but 'pseudo-secured'. This means that the primary good is only secured temporarily (if at all), as it is continuously under threat. Take, for instance, an individual who secures their primary good of Relatedness by acting in a controlling and violent manner towards an intimate partner. Relatedness may be 'pseudo-secured' as the relationship continues due to the partner's fear of leaving, however, the warm, affectionate aspects are unlikely to be fully realized. Importantly, where primary goods are only pseudo-secured, the individual is left feeling frustrated, meaning the likelihood that they will have a happy, meaningful, and fulfilling life is low [36].

The second obstacle, coherence, refers to the need for primary goods to be ordered and rationally related to each other. Where coherence is lacking, individuals feel frustrated and struggle to find meaning and purpose in life [40]. Primary goods can be related either horizontally or vertically [26]. Horizontal coherence refers to a harmonious relationship between primary goods, where they complement and enable each other. However, when primary goods are not horizontally coherent, conflict between goods can occur, leading to the use of inappropriate means. For example, an individual may place an equally high level of importance on the attainment of both Relatedness and Excellence in Agency. To attain Relatedness, they establish a close and secure romantic relationship. However, this conflicts with the attainment of Excellence in Agency; if they have no other opportunities to exert their autonomy and independence, they may behave violently towards their intimate partner to gain this sense of power and control.

Comparatively, vertical coherence refers to ranking of primary goods according to their degree of importance [40]. The level of importance assigned to primary goods differs according to the person's preferences, as well as social and cultural norms, and is closely linked to the conceptualization of their personal identity. An individual's behavior should be informed by the degree of importance assigned to each, with primary goods rated as highly important given the most amount of attention. For example, someone who rates Inner Peace as most important is going to be unhappy if they instead attain Excellence in Work by working in an environment that causes a high degree of stress. If there is a paucity of vertical coherence, the individual feels unfulfilled and lacks a sense of meaning and purpose in life. Ward and Stewart [26] suggests this leads to the neglect of long-term goals, in favor of immediate gratification. Thus, continuing with the previous example, the individual could attempt to relieve the stress from work (and attain Inner Peace) by expressing their emotions through negative means (i.e., acting violently, either towards themselves or others).

Although the level of importance differs for each primary good, all primary goods must be attained (to some degree) for a happy and meaningful life [27]. Neglecting or failing to strive for a primary good is considered a lack of scope [41]. Whilst disinterest plays a role in the neglect of primary goods, problems in capacity (i.e., skills and resources) tend to be the leading cause of a lack of scope. For instance, an individual with poor communication skills would (at a minimum) have difficulty securing the primary goods of Relatedness and Community. As a result of the frustration caused, the individual may engage in violent behavior. Supporting this, a review of factors for perpetrating IPV found 48% of studies included communication difficulties as a common motive [42].

The final obstacle, lack of capacity, refers to an individual experiencing a deficit in their internal skills and abilities (cognitive, psychological, and/or behavioral) or external resources (i.e., opportunities and/or environments) necessary to attain their primary goods. It must be noted that capacity issues are synonymous with 'criminogenic needs' (as used in the wider literature [40]). Both internal and external capacity issues have been identified as causal factors in violent behavior [43]. Regarding internal capacity issues, violent behavior has been associated with (among other factors) poor emotion regulation abilities, oppositional behaviors, impulsivity, callous-unemotional traits, and mental illness [44,45]. Furthermore, poverty, lack of employment opportunities, witnessing familial conflict, exposure to community violence and having antisocial peers are examples of external capacity issues that can lead an individual to engage in violent behavior [46,47].

When an individual experiences internal and external capacity issues, this can prevent the attainment of primary goods through prosocial means. For instance, past research has suggested that individuals exhibiting oppositional behaviors have difficulty securing and maintaining employment [48], supporting the assumption that attainment of Excellence in Work is prevented by issues in internal capacity. Concerning external capacity issues, if an individual lives in an area where competition for employment is high, this can equally prevent attainment of Excellence in Work. If the individual is unable to find a prosocial means of achieving the primary goods, then antisocial means may be used in an attempt to fulfil these (e.g., joining a gang as a form of 'employment' [49]). This highlights that internal and external capacity issues can prevent attainment of primary goods, with failure leading to frustration and engagement in violence. Critically, an individual is most vulnerable to engaging in violence if they are exposed to multiple internal and external capacity issues [40].

3. Good Lives Model: A Framework for Violence Intervention

As an intervention framework, the GLM guides the development and implementation of evidence-based interventions by emphasizing adherence to GLM-consistent treatment assumptions [50]. The key assumption guiding GLM-consistent treatment is that dual-focus should be placed on promoting prosocial attainment of primary goods, whilst also reducing risk of violence [51]. The GLM is considered a strengths-based approach to violence intervention, whereby an individual's personal strengths, goals, and interests are considered and built upon. When support is given to attain primary goods, through enhancing internal skills and providing external opportunities and resources, this should simultaneously lead to a reduction in violent behavior. Ultimately, the aim of GLM-consistent treatment is to help individuals attain a 'good life': one which is both personally meaningful and socially acceptable [39].

This differs from risk-based approaches to violence intervention, as GLM-consistent treatment aims to replace what is lost when violent behavior ceases [50]. Take the analogy of a pincushion: if all pins are removed but there is nothing to replace them, then the cushion will be left full of holes. Similarly, if all risk factors (e.g., spending time with antisocial peers and engaging in substance misuse) are removed, without providing an alternative means of achieving primary goods, an individual will be left frustrated and unhappy [26]. Therefore, in addition to reducing violent behavior, supporting the successful attainment of primary goods through prosocial means should lead to improvements in an individual's overall well-being, with increased happiness and reduced frustration [27].

When providing GLM-consistent treatment to an individual exhibiting violent behavior, a clinical interview should initially be conducted with the client. For examples of questions used to guide the clinical interview, see Griffin and Wylie [52]. The aims of the clinical interview are to explore: (a) how primary goods were sought at the time of the violent episode(s), (b) what secondary goods were used to attain primary goods, (c) issues in means, scope, coherence, and capacity, (d) personal strengths (i.e., internal capacities) and means (i.e., external capacities) currently available to the client, and (e) contexts or environments the client will be exposed to throughout and following an intervention. This leads to the creation of an individualized action plan, termed a 'Good Lives Plan', which highlights the skills and resources that should be targeted during interventions to enable attainment of primary goods through prosocial means. Collaboration between the client and therapist is essential in the creation of a Good Lives Plan. This encourages focus on primary goods of importance to the individual and enables the formulation of personally meaningful goals (short, medium, and long term), ensuring the Good Lives Plan is motivational and achievable [39].

As an intervention framework, the GLM can wrap around existing evidence-based treatment programs. Therefore, a Good Lives Plan guides which treatment programs (e.g., Cognitive Behavioral Therapy, Functional Family Therapy, substance use groups), skills programs (e.g., educational programs, apprenticeships) and/or external resources (e.g., access to employment opportunities, health care, prosocial support networks) would be most appropriate for a client to receive. Furthermore, the GLM informs how these treatment programs should be implemented, with considerations given to the ethics, goal formation, language used, and therapist characteristics. Specifically, GLM-consistent treatment should emphasize the client's agency, autonomy, and dignity [31]. In addition, GLM-consistent treatment should also utilize approach (rather than avoidance) goals, which highlight that a future without violence is both achievable and attractive [39]. Consistent with a strengths-based approach, the GLM expects positively framed language to be used throughout treatment programs, whereby focus is placed on skills rather than deficits of a client [26]. Finally, therapists are encouraged to demonstrate empathy, warmth, and respect towards clients, which aids in building a strong therapeutic alliance [53].

The GLM is frequently used to guide offender intervention world-wide and has been applied to numerous offending typologies including sexual offences, IPV, gang membership, and general violence [49,54–56]. A systematic review found GLM-consistent interventions were at least as effective as standard relapse prevention programs [57]. Specifically, pre-post measures of psychometric change did not differ between GLM-consistent and relapse prevention interventions [58,59]. In addition, clients that received GLM-consistent treatment report reduced feelings of shame, hopelessness, and defensiveness, and increased optimism for the future, confidence, perspective-taking ability, trust of others, and self-awareness [60,61]. Furthermore, in a case study, Whitehead et al. [55] discussed a high-risk violent offender who had received a GLM-consistent intervention. The client was supported to attain their primary goods, including engaging in education, pursuing new leisure activities, and maintaining a committed relationship. At a six-year follow-up, the client had not committed any further offences and had reduced engagement with street gang peers [62]. Of note, the client had previously received two intensive risk-oriented interventions but had continued to recidivate. This demonstrates that the GLM-consistent intervention was more successful in reducing violent behavior than risk-based interventions.

Findings from the only randomized control trial to date suggest participants who received GLM-consistent interventions demonstrated a greater motivation to desist from offending (as rated by therapists), had increased treatment engagement, and were more willing to disclose any lapses in behavior than participants that received standard relapse prevention treatment [63]. Whilst this supports the use of GLM-consistent interventions, it must be noted that the evidence-base remains in its infancy and primarily focuses on interventions for sexual offending. Critically, as the GLM is the preferred framework for offender intervention in one third of programs in the USA and half of programs in Canada [64], it is expected that the research base regarding the effectiveness of GLM-consistent interventions will rapidly increase in the coming years.

4. Interagency Collaboration in Violence Intervention

Clients with a history of violent behavior often present with multiple internal and external obstacles that prevent attainment of primary goods through prosocial means [49]. The clients' needs span multiple domains (e.g., individual, family, peer, education, and community), meaning multifaceted solutions are required to support attainment of primary goods and reduce violent recidivism [65]. Effectively responding to the complex and interrelated needs of a client is beyond the scope of a single organization and has led to the call for interagency collaboration [66]. To clarify, in this paper, interagency collaboration is defined as the coordinated effort of various organizations in achieving a common goal, such as violence prevention [67].

The primary benefit of interagency collaboration is improved access to different expertise and resources, which enables a holistic approach to client care [68]. With the common goal being the reduction of violence, a variety of agencies have specialized skills that could increase the possibility of fulfilling this. Social services, healthcare, criminal justice systems, education, community services, and psychological therapists are just a few examples of specialist agencies that can play a key role in violence interventions. For example, social services have the resources and expertise available to provide family-based interventions, healthcare services can support physical wellbeing, and community services can support the attainment of practical needs (e.g., housing and employment).

To date, research has suggested that interagency collaboration is crucial in both reducing rates of incarceration and preventing violent recidivism [65]. Interventions which utilize interagency collaboration also have higher retention rates and clients demonstrating reduced reliance on substances [69]. Furthermore, parents report their child exhibits improved attitudes, reduced risk-taking and antisocial behavior, and improved family relationships after receiving treatment from youth offending programs with interagency collaboration [70]. Regarding violence intervention specifically, programs with interagency collaboration have led to a significant reduction in violent behavior [71]. For example, the Cincinnati Initiative to Reduce Violence (CIRV) involved an interagency collaboration between law enforcement, community services (e.g., street advocates), healthcare professionals, researchers, and businesses, resulting in a 61% reduction in violence. The impact of CIRV on reducing gang-related homicides and violent firearm offences was maintained for a 42-month follow-up time [72].

Critically, most research on the effectiveness of programs incorporating interagency collaboration suffers from a lack of control group. Overcoming this, Pullman et al. [73] compared youth offenders receiving mental health treatment with an interagency collaboration to a control group of youth offenders receiving mental health treatment without interagency collaboration. Compared to the control, youth offenders receiving interagency treatment were less likely to reoffend and spent less time incarcerated. In addition, significant improvements in functioning at home, school, and in the community, and reduced emotional and behavioral problems were experienced by youth offenders receiving interagency treatment. With the growth in research supporting interagency collaboration, this is now advocated as 'best-practice' for offender interventions, including violence prevention, internationally [74,75].

Despite this, Statham [76] purports that interagency collaboration is "not inherently a good thing" (p. 4). Specifically, when interagency collaboration is done well, the effectiveness of offender interventions improves. However, when interagency collaboration is poorly implemented, this can have a negative impact on outcomes of offender interventions [77]. A multitude of barriers have been identified which can prevent the effective implementation of interventions with an interagency collaboration. According to Cooper et al. [78], the most common barriers are poor communication and trust between agencies, confidentiality issues, and a lack of time and resources. In addition, fundamental differences in values, goals, and methods between agencies can significantly hinder the implementation and success of collaborative approaches to offender intervention [79]. For instance, in their evaluation of an interagency approach to violence intervention (incorporating police, social services and community organizations), Gripp et al. [71] found initial resistance among police towards the collaboration, with officers describing the initiative as "another hug-a-thug program" (p. 50).

Whilst barriers do exist and are important to recognize, there are several factors that can facilitate good interagency collaboration. Firstly, having an open line of communication can improve relationships and trust between agencies. Researchers suggest monthly meetings between agencies to discuss clients' progress and share information are key for establishing positive communication [77]. Appointing a project manager can further enhance communication by balancing multiple and, at times, conflictual points of view [71]. Furthermore, joint training opportunities can improve understanding of the overarching goals, philosophy, and procedures surrounding offender intervention programs, emphasizing the benefits of working collaboratively [80]. In addition, procedures regarding information sharing and confidentiality need to be made clear to all agencies and clients at the beginning of an offender intervention program [81]. When implemented properly, interagency collaborations are the most effective means of delivering a holistic and responsive service for clients engaging in interventions for violent behavior [28].

5. Interagency Collaboration in Good Lives Interventions

The GLM is one intervention framework that emphasizes and, to some degree, relies on support from interagency collaborations. With 11 primary goods covering a diversity of needs, helping a client to attain these would be beyond the expertise of a single agency. As all primary goods must be attained for a fulfilling and meaningful life [27], it is important that some are not neglected simply due to the expertise of the agency leading client care. For example, psychological services have the expertise and resources available to support clients in overcoming internal capacity obstacles (e.g., developing coping strategies, improving mental health and interpersonal skills). This can lead to the attainment of primary goods such as Inner Peace and Relatedness. However, when working independently, psychological services may not have the resources available to target all external obstacles (e.g., access to housing, education, and employment opportunities), which can lead to some primary goods being neglected. When working in partnership with other agencies, this gap in expertise and resources can be filled.

At first glance, it may seem obvious which agencies are needed to aid in the attainment of primary goods. For instance, the primary good of Life (i.e., possessing the basic needs for survival, physical well-being, and functioning) may be attained by support from health care (i.e., ensuring physical well-being) or housing (i.e., shelter as a basic need) services. However, it is important to look beyond this over-simplified classification of the primary goods and focus on the capacity obstacles each client is experiencing. Specifically, a client with depression may neglect to care for their physical well-being [82], preventing the attainment of Life. Therefore, this client would require support from agencies specializing in psychological therapies. This demonstrates the need for an individualized approach to violence intervention, with the degree of input from different agencies dependent on the individuals' Good Lives Plan.

When developing a violence intervention consistent with GLM assumptions, it is recommended that these steps are first followed:

(1) Identify agencies that would be beneficial to a collaborative approach. This could include psychological services, criminal justice services (e.g., probation, police, prison service), social services, education, housing, community organizations (e.g., employment/volunteering), or healthcare. As explained above, the degree of input required from each agency will differ depending on the client, with some clients needing a great deal of input from agencies, whilst others require little to no support. However, establishing good contact with a variety of agencies during the planning stages of an intervention will prevent any delay in client care.

(2) Provide interagency training explaining the assumptions of the GLM and goals of GLM-consistent interventions. Some agencies may be used to a risk approach to

violence intervention with avoidance-focused goals. It is important to emphasize in training that the GLM advocates the use of a strengths-based method, with approach-focused goals, and that this must remain consistent throughout the intervention.

(3) Embed a project lead to enhance communication and balance differing values and goals across agencies. The project lead should have expertise in the GLM to ensure that the intervention planning remains consistent with the assumptions of the GLM (i.e., focus on developing strengths, overcoming internal and external capacity obstacles, ensuring a well-rounded intervention incorporating all primary goods).

(4) Discuss confidentiality and information sharing issues/caveats and establish the procedures surrounding this.

Regarding the implementation of a GLM-consistent intervention with clients, it is recommended that this procedure is followed:

(1) Therapist specializing in the GLM conducts a clinical interview with the client exploring: (a) how primary goods were sought at the time of the violent episode(s), (b) what secondary goods were used to attain primary goods, (c) issues in means, scope, coherence, and capacity, (d) personal strengths (i.e., internal capacities) and means (i.e., external capacities) currently available to the client, and (e) contexts or environments the client will be exposed to throughout and following an intervention.

(2) In collaboration with the client, create a Good Lives Plan. This should be a strengths-focused action plan, incorporating an individual's goals that, if attained, would enable them to have a meaningful and happy life without the need to offend. A Good Lives Plan should be realistic and achievable; whilst long-term goals are important, incremental attainable steps should be included. This enables a sense of achievement and supports motivation to pursue longer-term goals. Furthermore, the clients support networks, environments, and capacity should be considered when developing a Good Lives Plan, as this will impact upon how attainable goals are.

(3) Based on the clients' Good Lives Plan, the therapist formulates an intervention strategy. This highlights the obstacles (both internal and external) preventing effective attainment of primary goods that need targeting during an intervention and highlights which agencies would be best placed to support the client with each obstacle. It is likely that support from multiple agencies will be needed. For instance, a client may be unable to attain the primary good of Life due to homelessness, meaning support from community housing services is necessary. In addition, they may engage in violent behavior to express negative emotions (i.e., attain Inner Peace), which indicates support is needed from psychological services.

(4) Regular meetings between agencies (at least once a month) should be implemented to ensure continuity in client care and sharing of information regarding progress. Critically, as a client's goals or obstacles can change, be attained, or overcome, a Good Lives Plan should be viewed as a dynamic and adaptable tool that guides and supports therapeutic work. As such, good communication between agencies involved in client care is vital.

Interagency collaboration provides a well-rounded approach to violence intervention, with the provision of expertise and resources beyond that which a single agency could offer. Ultimately, this will further support the client in overcoming various internal and external capacity obstacles which can lead to their violent behavior. This will simultaneously lead to a reduction in the criminogenic needs of the client, reducing their likelihood of engaging in violence in the future [50]. Importantly, this will also support the attainment of each of the 11 primary goods, which will enable the client to have a life which is both personally meaningful and socially acceptable [39].

6. Conclusions

The response to violence has primarily been risk-focused and fragmented [4]. Theorists have argued that risk-focused frameworks have reached a "glass-ceiling", whereby further refining of interventions will not equate to reductions in reoffending [83]. As such, strengths-based approaches to violence intervention, including the GLM, are growing in popularity. The GLM recognizes the complexity of human behavior, suggesting violence occurs due to obstacles (internal and external) experienced in the pursuit of primary goods. By supporting clients to overcome these obstacles and effectively attain their primary goods, the GLM assumes that this will simultaneously lead to a reduction in violent behavior.

As each client will face various internal and external obstacles, interagency collaborations can provide the skills and resources necessary to assist in overcoming these, enabling the attainment of primary goods through prosocial means. Whilst barriers have been highlighted in past research [78], several recommendations can be made to support the implementation of an effective interagency collaboration. These include embedding a project lead to support good communication between agencies, holding regular interagency meetings, providing regular interagency training, defining the role each agency plays in client care, and establishing information sharing and confidentiality procedures at an early stage [77]. If done well, interagency collaboration can support clients to have a happy and meaningful life, free from violence.

Funding: This research received no external funding.

Institutional Review Board Statement: Not applicable, no participants involved, theoretical only.

Informed Consent Statement: Not applicable, no participants involved, theoretical only.

Conflicts of Interest: The author declares no conflict of interest.

References

1. World Health Organization. Injuries and Violence: The Facts. 2014. Available online: https://apps.who.int/iris/handle/10665/149798 (accessed on 23 June 2021).
2. United Nations Office on Drugs and Crime. Available online: https://www.unodc.org (accessed on 23 June 2021).
3. World Health Organization. Violence: A Public Health Priority. 1996. Available online: https://apps.who.int/iris/handle/10665/179463 (accessed on 23 June 2021).
4. World Health Organization. World Report on Violence and Health. 2002. Available online: http://apps.who.int/iris/bitstream/handle/10665/42495/9241545615_eng.pdf?sequence=1 (accessed on 23 June 2021).
5. World Health Organization. Violence against Women. 2021. Available online: https://www.who.int/news-room/fact-sheets/detail/violence-against-women (accessed on 23 June 2021).
6. Hillis, S.; Mercy, J.; Amobi, A.; Kress, H. Global prevalence of past-year violence against children: A systematic review and minimum estimates. *Pediatrics* **2016**, *137*, 1–22. [CrossRef]
7. Spencer, C.; Mallory, A.B.; Cafferky, B.M.; Kimmes, J.G.; Beck, A.R.; Stith, S.M. Mental health factors and intimate partner violence perpetration and victimization: A meta-analysis. *Psychol. Violence* **2019**, *9*, 1–17. [CrossRef]
8. Black, M.C. Intimate partner violence and adverse health consequences: Implications for clinicians. *Anal. Rev.* **2011**, *5*, 428–439. [CrossRef]
9. Adams, E.B.; Morris, P.K.; Maguire, E.R. The impact of gangs on community life in Trinidad. *Race Justice* **2018**, *1*, 1–24. [CrossRef]
10. Nofziger, S.; Kurtz, D. Violent lives: A lifestyle model linking exposure to violence to juvenile violent offending. *J. Res. Crime Delinq.* **2005**, *42*, 3–26. [CrossRef]
11. Rowan, Z.R.; Schubert, C.A.; Loughran, T.A.; Mulvey, E.P.; Pardini, D.A. Proximal predictors of gun violence among adolescent males involved in crime. *Law Hum. Behav.* **2019**, *43*, 250–262. [CrossRef]
12. Augustyn, M.B.; Thornberry, T.P.; Krohn, M.D. Gang membership and pathways to maladaptive parenting. *J. Res. Adolesc.* **2014**, *24*, 252–267. [CrossRef]
13. Nydegger, L.A.; DiFranceisco, W.; Quinn, K.; Dickson-Gomez, J. Gender norms and age-disparate sexual relationships as predictors of intimate partner violence, sexual violence, and risky sex among adolescent gang members. *J. Urban Health* **2017**, *94*, 266–275. [CrossRef] [PubMed]
14. DeLisi, M.; Drury, A.J.; Elbert, M.J. Do behavioral disorders render gang status spurious? New insights. *Int. J. Law Psychiatry* **2019**, *62*, 117–124. [CrossRef] [PubMed]
15. Forke, C.M.; Myers, R.K.; Fein, J.A.; Catallozzi, M.; Localio, A.R.; Wiebe, D.J.; Grisso, J.A. Witnessing intimate partner violence as a child: How boys and girls model their parents' behaviors in adolescence. *Child Abus. Neglec.* **2018**, *84*, 241–252.
16. Klein, M.W.; Maxson, C.L. *Street Gang Patterns and Policies*; Oxford University Press: Oxford, UK, 2006.
17. Muftić, L.R.; Smith, M. Sex, parental incarceration, and violence perpetration among a sample of young adults. *J. Interpers. Violence* **2018**, *33*, 316–338. [CrossRef]
18. Alleyne, E.; Wood, J.L. Gang-related crime: The social, psychological and behavioral correlates. *Psychol. Crime Law* **2013**, *19*, 611–627. [CrossRef]

19. O'Brien, K.; Daffern, M.; Chu, C.M.; Thomas, S.D.M. Youth gang affiliation, violence, and criminal activities: A review of motivational, risk, and protective factors. *Aggress. Violent Behav.* **2013**, *18*, 417–425. [CrossRef]

20. Ttofi, M.M.; Farrington, D.P.; Lösel, F. School bullying as a predictor of violence later in life: A systematic review and meta-analysis of prospective longitudinal studies. *Aggress. Violent Behav.* **2012**, *17*, 405–418. [CrossRef]

21. Rosenbaum, J. Educational and criminal justice outcomes 12 years after school suspension. *Youth Soc.* **2020**, *52*, 515–547. [CrossRef] [PubMed]

22. Savage, J.; Ellis, S.K. Academic achievement, school attachment, and school problems in the differential etiology of violence. *J. Dev. Life Course Criminol.* **2019**, *5*, 243–265. [CrossRef]

23. Volungis, A.M.; Goodman, K. School violence prevention: Teachers establishing relationships with students using counseling strategies. *Sage Open* **2017**, *7*, 1–11. [CrossRef]

24. Franzese, R.J.; Menard, S.; Weiss, A.J.; Covey, H.C. Adolescent exposure to violence and adult violent victimization and offending. *Crim. Justice Rev.* **2017**, *42*, 42–57. [CrossRef]

25. Public Health England. A Whole-System Multi-Agency Approach to Serious Violence Prevention. 2019. Available online: https://assets.publishing.service.gov.uk/government/uploads/system/uploads/attachment_data/file/862794/multi-agency_approach_to_serious_violence_prevention.pdf (accessed on 23 June 2021).

26. Ward, T.; Stewart, C. The relationship between human needs and criminogenic needs. *Psychol. Crime Law* **2003**, *9*, 219–224. [CrossRef]

27. Ward, T.; Maruna, S. *Rehabilitation: Beyond the Risk Paradigm*; Routledge: Oxford, UK, 2007.

28. Banks, D.; Dutch, N.; Wang, K. Collaborative efforts to improve system response to families who are experiencing child maltreatment and domestic violence. *J. Interpers. Violence* **2008**, *23*, 876–902. [CrossRef]

29. Ward, T. Good Lives and the rehabilitation of offenders: Promises and problems. *Aggress. Violent Behav.* **2002**, *7*, 513–528. [CrossRef]

30. Laws, D.R.; Ward, T. *Desistance from Sex Offender: Alternatives to Throwing Away the Keys*; The Guildford Press: New York, NY, USA, 2011.

31. Ward, T.; Syversen, K. Human dignity and vulnerable agency: An ethical framework for forensic practice. *Aggress. Violent Behav.* **2009**, *14*, 94–105. [CrossRef]

32. Deci, E.L.; Ryan, R.M. The 'what' and 'why' of goal pursuits: Human needs and the self-determination of behavior. *Psychol. Inq.* **2000**, *11*, 227–268. [CrossRef]

33. Mallion, J.S. Application of Good Lives Model to Street Gang Members. Ph.D. Thesis, University of Kent, Canterbury, UK, 2021.

34. Alleyne, E.; Wood, J.L. Gang involvement: Psychological and behavioral characteristics of gang members, peripheral youth, and nongang youth. *Aggress. Behav.* **2010**, *36*, 423–436. [CrossRef]

35. Kloess, J.A.; Beech, A.R.; Harkins, L. Online child sexual exploitation: Prevalence, process, and offender characteristics. *Trauma Violence Abus.* **2014**, *15*, 126–139. [CrossRef] [PubMed]

36. Purvis, M. *Seeking a Good Life: Human Goods and Sexual Offending*; Lambert Academic Press: Chisinau, Moldova, 2010.

37. Higgins, G.E.; Piquero, N.L.; Piquero, A.R. General strain theory, peer rejection, and delinquency/crime. *Youth Soc.* **2011**, *43*, 1272–1297. [CrossRef]

38. Gannon, T.A.; King, T.; Miles, H.; Lockerbie, L.; Willis, G.M. Good Lives sexual offender treatment for mentally disordered offenders. *Br. J. Forensic Pract.* **2011**, *13*, 153–168. [CrossRef]

39. Ward, T.; Fortune, C.A. The Good Lives Model: Aligning risk reduction with promoting offenders' personal goals. *Eur. J. Probat.* **2013**, *5*, 29–46. [CrossRef]

40. Purvis, M.; Ward, T.; Willis, G. The Good Lives Model in practice: Offence pathways and case management. *Eur. J. Probat.* **2013**, *5*, 29–46. [CrossRef]

41. Chu, C.M.; Koh, L.L.; Zeng, G.; Teoh, J. Youth who sexual offended: Primary human goods and offense pathways. *Sex. Abus.* **2015**, *27*, 151–172. [CrossRef]

42. Langhinrichsen-Rohling, J.; McCullars, A.; Misra, T. Motivation for men and women's intimate partner violence perpetration: A comprehensive review. *Partn. Abus.* **2012**, *3*, 429–468. [CrossRef]

43. Bernat, D.H.; Oakes, M.; Pettingell, S.L.; Resnick, M. Risk and direct protective factors for youth violence: Results from the national longitudinal study of adolescent health. *Am. J. Prev. Med.* **2012**, *43*, 57–66. [CrossRef]

44. Romero-Martínez, Á.; Lila, M.; Moya-Albiol, L. The importance of impulsivity and attention switching deficits in perpetrators convicted for intimate partner violence. *Aggress. Behav.* **2019**, *45*, 129–138. [CrossRef]

45. Wood, J.L.; Kallis, C.; Coid, J.W. Differentiating gang members, gang affiliates and violent men on their psychiatric morbidity and traumatic experiences. *Psychiatry* **2017**, *80*, 221–235.

46. Dishion, T.J.; Véronneau, M.-H.; Myers, M. Cascading peer dynamics underlying the progression from problem behavior to violence in early to late adolescence. *Dev. Psychopathol.* **2010**, *22*, 603–619. [CrossRef]

47. Park, S.; Kim, S.-H. The power of family and community factors in predicting dating violence: A meta-analysis. *Aggress. Violent Behav.* **2018**, *40*, 19–28. [CrossRef]

48. Burke, J.D.; Rowe, R.; Boylan, K. Functional outcomes of child and adolescent oppositional defiant disorder symptoms in young adult men. *J. Child Psychol. Psychiatry* **2014**, *55*, 264–272. [CrossRef] [PubMed]

49. Mallion, J.S.; Wood, J.L. Good Lives Model and street gang membership: A review and application. *Aggress. Violent Behav.* **2020**, *52*, 1–11. [CrossRef]
50. Ward, T.; Yates, P.M.; Willis, G.M. The Good Lives Model and the Risk Need Responsivity Model: A response to Andrews, Bonta, and Wormith (2011). *Crim. Justice Behav.* **2012**, *39*, 94–110. [CrossRef]
51. Ward, T.; Gannon, T.A. Rehabilitation, etiology, and self-regulation: The comprehensive good lives model of treatment for sexual offenders. *Aggress. Violent Behav.* **2006**, *11*, 77–94. [CrossRef]
52. Griffin, M.L.; Wylie, H. The journey: G-map's adaptation of the Good Lives Model. In *The Good Lives Model for Adolescents Who Sexually Harm*; Print, B., Ward, T., Eds.; The Safer Society Press: Brandon, VT, USA, 2013; pp. 35–54.
53. Barnao, M.; Ward, T.; Robertson, P. The Good Lives Model: A new paradigm for forensic mental health. *Psychiatry Psychol. Law* **2015**, *23*, 288–301. [CrossRef]
54. Langlands, R.L.; Ward, T.; Gilchrist, E. Applying the Good Lives Model to male perpetrators of domestic violence. *Behav. Chang.* **2009**, *26*, 113–129. [CrossRef]
55. Whitehead, P.R.; Ward, T.; Collie, R.M. Time for a change: Applying the good lives model of rehabilitation to a high-risk violent offender. *Int. J. Offender Ther. Comp. Criminol.* **2007**, *51*, 578–598. [CrossRef] [PubMed]
56. Willis, G.M.; Prescott, D.S.; Yates, P.M. The Good Lives Model (GLM) in theory and practice. *Sex. Abus. Aust. New Zealand* **2013**, *5*, 3–9.
57. Mallion, J.S.; Wood, J.L.; Mallion, A. Systematic review of 'Good Lives' assumptions and interventions. *Aggress. Violent Behav.* **2020**, *55*, 1–17. [CrossRef]
58. Harkins, L.; Flak, V.E.; Beech, A.R.; Woodhams, J. Evaluation of a community-based sex offender treatment program using a good lives model approach. *Sex. Abus.* **2012**, *24*, 519–543. [CrossRef]
59. Barnett, G.D.; Manderville-Norden, R.; Rakestrow, J. The Good Lives Model or relapse prevention: What works better in facilitating change? *Sex. Abus.* **2014**, *26*, 3–33. [CrossRef]
60. Leeson, S.; Adshead, M. The response of adolescents and practitioners to a Good Lives approach. In *The Good Lives Model for Adolescents who Sexually Harm*; Print, B., Ward, T., Eds.; The Safer Society Press: Brandon, VT, USA, 2013; pp. 183–193.
61. Ward, M.; Attwell, P. Evaluation of two community outreach forensic psychological services. *J. Forensic Pract.* **2014**, *16*, 312–326. [CrossRef]
62. Willis, G.M.; Ward, T. The Good Lives Model: Does it work? Preliminary evidence. In *What Works in Offender Rehabilitation: An Evidence-Based Approach to Assessment and Treatment*; Craig, A., Dixon, L., Gannon, T.A., Eds.; John Wiley & Sons: Hoboken, NJ, USA, 2013; pp. 305–317.
63. Mann, R.E.; Webster, S.D.; Schofield, C.; Marshall, W.L. Approach versus avoidance goals in relapse prevention with sexual offenders. *Sex. Abus. J. Res. Treat.* **2004**, *16*, 65–75. [CrossRef]
64. McGrath, R.J.; Cumming, G.F.; Burchard, B.L.; Zeoli, S.; Ellerby, L. Current Practices and Emerging Trends in Sexual Abuser Management. 2009. Available online: http://www.robertmcgrath.us/files/6414/3204/5288/2009_Safer_Society_North_American_Survey.pdf (accessed on 24 June 2021).
65. Rocha, P. Meeting criminogenic needs to reduce recidivism: The diversion of vulnerable offenders from the criminal justice system into care. *Int. J. Law Political Sci.* **2019**, *13*, 831–837.
66. Nicholson, D.; Artz, S.; Armitage, A.; Fagan, J. Working relationships and outcomes in multidisciplinary collaborative practice settings. In *Child and Youth Care Forum*; Kluwer Academic Publishers-Plenum Publishers: Norwell, MA, USA, 2000; Volume 29, pp. 39–73.
67. Fletcher, B.W.; Lehman, W.E.; Wexler, H.K.; Melnick, G.; Taxman, F.S.; Young, D.W. Measuring collaboration and integration activities in criminal justice and substance abuse treatment agencies. *Drug Alcohol Depend.* **2009**, *103*, 54–64. [CrossRef]
68. Strype, J.; Gundhus, H.I.; Egge, M.; Ødegård, A. Perceptions of interprofessional collaboration. *Prof. Prof.* **2014**, *4*, 1–16. [CrossRef]
69. Yatsco, A.J.; Champagne-Langabeer, T.; Holder, T.F.; Stotts, A.L.; Langabeer, J.R. Developing interagency collaboration to address the opioid epidemic: A scoping review of joint criminal justice and healthcare initiatives. *Int. J. Drug Policy* **2020**, *83*, 1–7. [CrossRef]
70. Oliver, C.; Mooney, A.; Statham, J. Integrated Working: A Review of the Evidence. 2010. Available online: https://dera.ioe.ac.uk/3674/1/Integrated_Working_A_Review_of_the_Evidence_report.pdf (accessed on 24 June 2021).
71. Gripp, C.; Jha, C.; Vaughn, P.E. Enhancing community safety through interagency collaboration: Lessons from Connecticut's Project Longevity. *J. Law Med. Ethics* **2020**, *48*, 47–54. [CrossRef] [PubMed]
72. Engel, R.S.; Tillyer, M.S.; Corsaro, N. Reducing gang violence using focused deterrence: Evaluating the Cincinnati Initiative to Reduce Violence (CIRV). *Justice Q.* **2013**, *30*, 403–439. [CrossRef]
73. Pullmann, M.D.; Kerbs, J.; Koroloff, N.; Veach-White, E.; Gaylor, R.; Sieler, D. Juvenile offenders with mental health needs: Reducing recidivism using wraparound. *Crime Delinq.* **2006**, *52*, 375–397. [CrossRef]
74. Department of Health. Equity and Excellence: Liberating the NHS. 2010. Available online: https://navigator.health.org.uk/theme/equity-and-excellence-liberating-nhs-white-paper?gclid=Cj0KCQjw2tCGBhCLARIsABJGmZ64nHDSPA_xpf34-fSZUrFiIWuTq6gyHyRUKM8tv3mXYkENJQAY7UQaAioHEALw_wcB (accessed on 23 June 2021).
75. Murray, S.; Powell, A. *Domestic Violence: Australian Public Policy*; Australian Scholarly Publishing: Victoria, Australia, 2012.
76. Statham, J. A Review of International Evidence on Interagency Working, to Inform the Development of Children's Services Committees in Ireland. 2011. Available online: https://www.lenus.ie/handle/10147/315237 (accessed on 24 June 2021).

77. Stewart, S.L. Enacting entangled practice: Interagency collaboration in domestic and family violence work. *Violence Women* **2020**, *26*, 191–212. [CrossRef]
78. Cooper, M.; Evans, Y.; Pybis, J. Interagency collaboration in children and young people's mental health: A systematic review of outcomes, facilitating factors and inhibiting factors. *Child Care Health Dev.* **2015**, *42*, 325–342. [CrossRef] [PubMed]
79. Lamberti, J.S. Preventing criminal recidivism through mental health and criminal justice collaboration. *Psychiatr. Serv.* **2016**, *67*, 1206–1212. [CrossRef]
80. Noonan, P.M.; McCall, Z.A.; Zheng, C.; Gaumer Erickson, A.S. An analysis of collaboration in a state-level interagency transition team. *Career Dev. Transit. Except. Individ.* **2012**, *35*, 143–154. [CrossRef]
81. Green, B.L.; Rockhill, A.; Burns, S. The role of interagency collaboration for substance-abusing families involved with child welfare. *Child Welf.* **2008**, *1*, 29–61.
82. Kessing, D.; Denollet, J.; Widdershoven, J.; Kupper, N. Self-care and health-related quality of life in chronic heart failure: A longitudinal analysis. *Eur. J. Cardiovasc. Nurs.* **2017**, *16*, 605–613. [CrossRef] [PubMed]
83. Porporino, F.J. Bringing sense and sensitivity to corrections: From programmes to 'fix' offenders to services to support desistance. In *What Else Works? Creative Work with Offenders*; Brayford, J., Cowe, F., Deering, J., Eds.; Routledge: Oxford, UK, 2010; pp. 61–87.

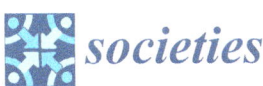

societies

MDPI

Article

Where You From? Examining the Relationship between Gang Migrants and Gang-Related Homicide

Daniel Scott

Department of Social Sciences, Texas A&M International University, Laredo, TX 78041, USA; daniel.scott@tamiu.edu

Abstract: Research has frequently focused on the increased likelihood of violence and homicide among gang-involved individuals, as well as on the factors that contribute to this violence. Such work has examined the relationship between immigration and the frequency of crime, as well. However, there is a dearth of research examining the likelihood of gang-related homicide and the presence of both gang migrants from within the U.S. and those from abroad in a given community. The current paper utilizes National Youth Gang Survey data to examine the relationship between law enforcement perceptions of gang migrants in their jurisdiction and the frequency of gang-related homicide. The results reveal that gang-related homicides have a significant and negative association with the presence of gang migrants. These findings have important policy implications for understanding and addressing serious gang violence and homicide at the community level.

Keywords: gang migrants; policing gangs; homicide; violence; prevention; collaboration

Citation: Scott, D. Where You From? Examining the Relationship between Gang Migrants and Gang-Related Homicide. *Societies* **2022**, *12*, 48. https://doi.org/10.3390/soc12020048

Academic Editors: Jaimee Mallion and Erika Gebo

Received: 7 February 2022
Accepted: 10 March 2022
Published: 12 March 2022

Publisher's Note: MDPI stays neutral with regard to jurisdictional claims in published maps and institutional affiliations.

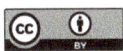

1. Introduction

Research has regularly revealed that gang members are more likely to become involved in crime and violence [1], as well as that gang members are more likely to engage in homicide. Due to this consistent relationship between gang involvement and violence, scholarship has examined specific characteristics of gangs and their members in order to improve comprehension of gang member criminality [2–4]. One area in which very little recent work has been conducted is on gang migrants from inside and outside of the United States.[1] Work conducted by Maxson (1997) revealed that gang migrants move for a variety of reasons, with the most frequent reason for moving being social [5]. Additional work has examined gang growth and migration in select jurisdictions in the United States, with varying results [6–9]. However, little work has examined the relationship between gang migrants and serious crime, including homicide.

Research has examined the relationship between immigration and crime with mixed results. While there are works that have found a significant and positive relationship between immigration and crime, suggesting that immigration brings with it an increased likelihood of crime in a community [10], most research has either found no significant relationship between immigration and crime [11] or a significant and negative association [12,13]. Scholarship examining immigration and gangs has revealed that in select areas, immigrants are more likely to join gangs [1]; however, this does not necessarily mean gangs with immigrants are likely to commit more crime. In fact, Duran's (2018) work highlights high levels of disproportionate minority contact with the system in areas close to the border. He specifically argues that the practices of "White Diversion" and "Minority Delinquentization" are occurring, and that disproportionate minority contact coincides with increased gang involvement [14].

Research has not yet examined whether the presence of gang migrants impacts the likelihood of serious gang violence such as homicide, or whether areas where police report high concentrations of gang migrants contributing to gang violence influence the probability of gang-related homicide. Given that research regularly finds a negative relationship between immigration and crime and a positive association between gang involvement and crime, it is critical to understand whether the concentration of gang member migrants in a community influences the likelihood of gang-related homicides. The current study contributes to this gap in the literature by analyzing the relationship between police reports of the percentage of gang member migrants in their jurisdiction, gang member migrants contributing to gang violence in their jurisdiction, and number of reported gang-related homicides. The results have implications for policy and can specifically inform approaches for communities to collaborate in order to address and prevent serious gang crime and violence more effectively.

The paper begins with a discussion of the relationship between immigration and crime, transitions into addressing work on gangs and crime, and concludes by addressing scholarship related to immigration and gangs. The paper then moves into the proposed hypotheses, analyses, and results and concludes with a discussion of the theoretical and policy implications. Specifically, the paper discusses the importance of police and community collaboration, as perceptions of serious violence and homicide vary between police, the public, and other data sources. These results have implications for collaborative community approaches seeking to reduce the likelihood of gang-related homicides and other serious gang violence, improve perceptions of safety in these communities, and foster positive relationships among community members.

2. Literature Review

2.1. Gang Violence and Homicide

Research regularly finds that gang members are more likely than non-gang members to participate in violence [1,15–17] and that gang members engage in violent behavior that is related to both gang and non-gang issues [18,19]. Research further reveals that gang violence may result from racial issues in combination with a need for group protection while trying to achieve control of territory in the same community [20–23]. Gang violence frequently occurs both between gangs [3,24] and within gangs [25]. More specifically, gangs regularly engage in violence due to internal gang conflict or rivalries as well as because of drugs, domestic violence, or robbery [26].

According to Decker and Curry (2002), gang homicides have unique characteristics that include the race of victim and perpetrator, drug involvement, victim–offender relationship, weapon use, spatial concentration, and sex. It is important to examine the likelihood of gang homicides among areas that police report gang migrants contributing to gang violence, as the nature of gang homicides are different than non-gang homicides [27–30]. Specifically, gang homicides often include incidents of both drive-by and walk-by shootings, homicide as a method of retaliation, and higher rates in concentrated spaces/areas of a community [3,15,31–33]. Similarly, Maxson et al. (1985) compared gang and non-gang homicides and found that gang homicides had a higher probability of involving gun use, vehicles, and occurring in public spaces [34]. Additionally, law enforcement has characterized gang homicides as having a greater likelihood of being violent and having more individuals involved as offender, accomplice, and victim. Furthermore, they found differences in a variety of individual-level characteristics, including age, ethnicity, and the relationship between involved parties.

Problems specific to gang homicides include the effect on families and communities [35]. Gangs influence the mentality of individual gang members in such a way that they may be willing to give their own life or engage in murder to show their commitment [36]. Research reveals that gang violence is impacted by multiple factors [37] which affect the likelihood of gang homicide, such as the frequency of gang membership in an area, population density, and social and economic deprivation [38]. Scholarship has not, however, specifically examined the influence that the presence of gang migrants has on the likelihood of gang-related homicide.

2.2. Gang Member Migration and Crime

Research has analyzed gang migrants both within the U.S. and abroad. Specifically, research has focused on why gang members move from one city to another and the impact of this on gang proliferation and crime. The occurrence of gang members migrating has been identified for several decades [39–42]. To this day, there has been very little work on gang migration, and most of this is community specific. Skolnick et al. (1988) found in their research with inmates and correctional staff that gangs expand to new areas to sell illegal drugs. Gangs in Milwaukee, for example, were primarily an outgrowth of Milwaukee, with only a small portion of the gang members coming from the Chicago area [6]. Although there are cases of gang members or gangs migrating to different communities in Southern California, it is not common [8]. Arguably, most gangs are groups of youth that do not have the resources to establish themselves outside of their own turf. Research in Kenosha, Wisconsin highlights that although police perceive that gangs in the area are migrating from Chicago, most of the gangs and gang problems are occurring due to local economic and social issues [9]. Furthermore, research examining why gang members move reveals that while they move for a variety of reasons, including illegal attractions such as drug market expansion, the most frequent reasons for moving were social and family-related [5].

According to the NYGS, the majority of jurisdictions reporting issues with gangs identified gang member migrants in the community [43]. Although the media often report migrating gang members as an issue that is getting worse, there is little data to support this, and there is little work on the topic. The general public views gang member migrants as contributing to gang violence, drugs, and conflict [44,45]. Research suggests that street gangs are connected to gangs in different communities due to gang migration [46]; additional work has revealed a relationship between gang migration and heightened gang activity, violent crime, and drug crime [47]. Other work, however, is contradictory, revealing a lack of significant association between gang member migrants and gang-related crimes [43].

Gang members migrate for both illegitimate and legitimate reasons, with legitimate social reasons the most frequent rationale reported for gang member migration [5]. It is possible that international gang member migration is connected to the adoption of different gang styles instead of gang substance [22]. Specifically, McGuire (2006) argues that although gang members may move, it is possible that gang style and practices are migrating as well [48]. Conversely, there have been reports of gang members migrating to different cities in Canada [46]. This includes local Canadian gangs establishing themselves in various areas in Canada. Street gangs in Toronto have arrived from the United States and Jamaica, and work has revealed gangs that moved from smaller to larger areas in Canada. Additionally, local gangs have been established in multiple communities, and there have been reports of gangs migrating from the U.S. to major cities in Canada such as Toronto [46]. Gang member migration is therefore relatively common and occurs for a variety of reasons. Results are mixed on the relationship between gang member migrants and gang-related crime, with suggestions that gang members may move to expand criminal enterprises, while other work identifies moving for social reasons [5]. Little research has examined the relationship between gang migrants and serious gang crime such as homicide.

2.3. Immigration, Crime, and Gangs

Given that the current study examines gang migrants from inside and outside the United States, it is important to discuss the relationship between immigration and crime. Research examining the relationship between immigration and crime regularly finds no significant association or a negative association with criminal behavior [49–55]. For example, immigrant youth are more afraid of being victimized by someone with a weapon compared to non-immigrant youth [56]. This suggests that there is a negative relationship between low acculturation and a high level of fear towards crime.

Communities located on the border in Texas tend to have Latino homicide rates that are lower than 50% of those in communities located away from the border [57]. Interestingly, in analysis of homicides in El Paso, TX, Emerick et al. 2014 found no significant association between immigration and homicide; however, there was a significant and positive relationship between the percentage of Latinos and gang-related homicides. Research reveals lower levels of homicide in areas with higher immigrant concentration; however, when focusing specifically on gang-related homicides there is a significant and positive association with immigration [58]. Other research has revealed that expatriate Latinos living in the U.S. have an increased likelihood of cooperating with law enforcement compared to Latinos born in the U.S. [12]. However, Latinos that have experienced police assault or have gang-involved friends have a lower probability of cooperation with law enforcement. Other studies have revealed that foreign-born Latinos have an increased probability of cooperating with police compared to their U.S.-born counterparts, and that this is consistent even when examining violent gang crimes [13,59].

Borders have unique conditions that can contribute to the production of gangs that are different than gangs in other areas, such as a "bi-national barrio-prison-cartel hybrid" gang located in El Paso [60]. Due to the already large number of gang members in the area, there is a large recruitment pool for gangs to grow. The different methods utilized to identify gangs and gang members could lead to both over-policing and criminalization of young immigrants [61]. Research by Esbensen and Carson (2012) revealed that when determining the major characteristics of gang youth, immigrant status was not found to be one of them, especially during a youth's time in middle school. More specifically, youth who reported being born outside of the United States had a lower probability of being gang-involved when younger; however, once these youth turn 15, immigrant youth make up a noticeable portion of the gang youth in their sample.

Gang members born outside of the United States are less likely to participate in crime compared to gang members born in the United States [62]. However, gang-involved youth are found to be more likely to participate in delinquency compared to non-gang youth irrespective of whether or not they were born outside of the United States. Consistent with these findings, Valdez et al. (2009) examined 28 homicides with Mexican-American gang members and found no immigrant youth involvement. Although similarly aged immigrant youth lived in the same areas where the violent incidents occurred, their involvement in gangs and violence was minimal [63]. Conversely, Hollis (2018) found a significant and positive relationship between Latino immigration and a greater amount of crime; however, this relationship is specific to non-gang crime [64]. When examining gang crime specifically, there is no significant association with Latino immigration. These findings suggest that even though gangs and gang involvement increase the likelihood of violence, the presence of immigrants may aid in reducing this probability of gang violence.

3. Research Questions and Hypotheses

Although research has examined the relationship between immigration, gangs, and crime and gang migrants and crime, there has been little work that has specifically examined the relationship between gang migrants from within and outside the United States and gang violence, including gang-related homicide. Given the mixed and limited findings in the research examining immigration, gang migrants from inside and outside of the United States, and gang crime, the current study asks the following question:

1. What is the relationship between gang migrants and gang-related homicide? Specifically, this paper hypothesizes that:

a.   In jurisdictions where law enforcement reports that gang migrants from inside the United States significantly influence gang-related violence, gang related-homicides are less likely to occur;

b.   In jurisdictions where law enforcement reports that gang migrants from outside the United States significantly influence gang-related violence, gang-related homicides are less likely to occur;

c.   The greater the percentage of migrant gang members in a jurisdiction, the less likely gang-related homicides are to occur.

4. Data and Methods

4.1. Data Description

The current study utilizes data from the 2012 National Youth Gang Survey (NYGS), which was the last year in which the NYGS was distributed. The NYGS was originally implemented to assess the severity of gang issues in the United States by examining law enforcement perspectives on where gangs exist, the different characteristics they have, and how their behaviors vary across communities. The items utilized in the NYGS are supported by scholarship [65]. Data collection occurred through the distribution of surveys to various law enforcement jurisdictions across the U.S. Specifically, all departments in jurisdictions of at least 50,000 and all suburban counties were sent surveys. Rural jurisdictions provided their perspective as well; surveys were provided to a random sample of law enforcement offices in communities with populations between 2500 and 49,000, in addition to counties categorized as rural. The strategy resulted in a representative sample with an 85% response rate from law enforcement jurisdictions across the United States, making it a good fit for the present study. The data allow for the ability to examine gang related homicide frequencies across jurisdictions that report varying levels of issues of gang migrants from the law enforcement perspective.

4.2. Analytical Methods

The analyses for the current study included both bivariate and multivariate methods. Due to the use of a variety of variable types, including dichotomous and ordinal independent variables and a count dependent variable, one-way analysis of variance was utilized. This allowed for comparison of gang migrant characteristics with gang-related homicides in different jurisdictions. In order to account for additional variables and decreased spuriousness, multivariate analyses were utilized. Due to the skewed count level dependent variable, negative binomial regression was used. Additionally, in order to account for missing cases in the data, multiple imputation was utilized in STATA (Release 16). By utilizing multiple imputation, values are able to imputed in the data where limited information is provided. When using multiple imputation, the assumption is made that there is no relationship between the likelihood of missing data on one variable and the variable's real value [66,67].

4.3. Variables

The number of gang-related homicides in a jurisdiction during the past year that were reported by law enforcement was included as the dependent variable. The number of gang-related homicides in the last year was determined through surveys distributed to various law enforcement jurisdictions across the United States.

The analyses included three independent variables. First, law enforcement was asked to provide the percentage of gang migrants in their community that were gang members. This was a scale level variable from 0–4, where 1 = 1–25%, 2 = includes 26–50%, 3 = 51–75%, and 4 = 76–100%. Second, two dichotomous variables asking law enforcement whether either gang members migrating from outside the United States or gang members migrating from inside the United States were significantly contributing to gang violence in their jurisdiction were included as independent variables.

Various control variables were included in the analyses. The number of gang-related homicides may differ across regions due to variations in methods of gang member identification [68]; thus, different regions of the United States (Northeast, Midwest, West, and South) were included as control variables. Moreover, given the potential relationship between gang presence and homicides, both the number of gangs and number of gang members were included in the analyses. Additional control variables included jurisdiction population, the length of time measured in years that law enforcement have reported gang problems, and whether or not the jurisdiction has a gang unit. Lastly, variables measuring whether there was a greater amount of offending before an individual joined a gang and/or more offending once they were committed to a gang were included as control variables.

5. Results

The data in Table 1 includes descriptive information on the average number of gang-related homicides in relation to the control variables included in the analyses.

Table 1. Control Variables Descriptives (N = 859)[2].

Control Variables	Mean Gang-Related Homicides in Last Year
Number of Active Gangs (n = 859)	
1–10	0.72
11–20	2.1
21–30	4.2
31–40	5
41–50	11.1
<50	9.7
Mean Number of Active Gang Members (n = 657)	
1–100	0.6
101–200	1.24
201–300	2
301–400	2.4
401–500	4.97
<500	4.94
Mean Number of Years there has been a Gang Problem (n = 859)	
>1	1.12
1–10	1.56
11–20	2.21
21–30	3.04
31–40	4
41–50	6.77
<50	9.04
Average Jurisdiction Population (n = 859)	
>100,000	0.763
100,000–199,999	1.98
200,000–299,999	5.29
300,000–399,999	10.43
400,000–499,999	7.83
<500,000	13.81
Prior Level of Offending (n = 641)	
Yes	2.65
No	2.31
Subsequent Level of Offending (n = 795)	
Yes	3.3
No	0.65
Region (n = 859)	
Northeast	2.8
South	1.92
Midwest	4.42
West	2.97
Gang Unit (n = 616)	
Yes	4.33
No	2.88

When looking at the number of active gangs reported in a jurisdiction, the average number of gang homicides reported increases with the number of active gangs in a jurisdiction. The mean number of gang-related homicides peaks at about 50 active gangs. This is similar when looking at the number of active gang members. The mean number of gang-related homicides peaks at about 500 active gang members. The average number of gang-related homicides tends to increase with the number of years police report that gangs have been a problem. Similarly, the more populated an area is, the higher the average number of gang-related homicides. Jurisdictions that report increased levels of offending after gang joining report a higher number of gang-related homicides on average compared to jurisdictions that do not report increased levels of offending after gang joining. The data highlight regional variations in the average number of gang homicides; jurisdictions with gang units report a higher number of gang-related homicides on average compared to jurisdictions without a gang unit.

5.1. Bivariate Analyses

The results of the bivariate analyses between police perceptions of gang migrants influencing gang related violence, reported percentage of gang migrants in a jurisdiction, and gang related homicides are displayed in Table 2.

Table 2. One-Way ANOVA Results and Mean Frequency of Gang-Related Homicides (n = 741).

Gang Migrant and Immigrant Variables	
Percentage Gang Migrants	**Gang-Related Homicides**
0%	2.14
1–25%	3.54
26–50%	2.2
51–75%	0.373
76–100%	0.316
Influence Gang-Related Violence	
Gang Members from other U.S. Jurisdictions	
Yes	1.58
No	3.47
Gang Members from Jurisdictions Outside the U.S.	
Yes	3.18
No	2.84

The average number of gang-related homicides is over twice as high in jurisdictions that do not report gang migrants from other U.S. jurisdictions influencing violence compared to jurisdictions that do report this influence. Conversely, there is minimal difference in the average number of gang-related homicides reported in jurisdictions where police identify gang migrants from outside the U.S. influencing gang violence compared to those that do not. Lastly, when police report that the percentage of gang members in a jurisdiction is greater than 25%, the average number of gang-related homicides begins to decrease. The results of the bivariate analyses do not reveal any statistically significant findings; however, these findings highlight the need to conduct multivariate analyses in order to improve comprehension of the relationship between gang migration and gang-related homicides.

5.2. Multivariate Results

The results in Table 3 include two models; Model 1 includes police reporting on gang migrants from the U.S. contributing to gang related violence in their jurisdiction as an independent variable, and Model 1 include police reporting on gang migrants from outside the U.S. contributing to gang related violence in their jurisdiction.

The findings in Model 1 do not support the first hypothesis. There is a significant and negative association between reporting that gang migrants within the U.S. influence gang-related violence and gang-related homicides. Therefore, in jurisdictions where police report that gang migrants within the U.S. significantly influence gang related violence, gang-related homicides are significantly less likely to occur. Additional findings reveal a significant and positive association between the number of active gangs and gang-related homicides, and a significant and negative association between the number of active gang members and gang-related homicides. Furthermore, the number of years there has been a gang problem, jurisdiction population, and increased likelihood of offending upon gang joining were all significant and positively associated with the likelihood of gang-related homicides.

Table 3. Gang Migrants from Inside/Outside the United States and Gang-Related Homicides (n = 781).

Independent Variables	Model 1 I.R.R. (S.E.)	Model 2 I.R.R. (S.E.)
Gang Migrants from U.S.	0.675 * (0.107)	-
Gang Migrants from Outside of U.S.	-	0.737 (0.155)
Northeast	1.51 † (0.3605)	1.53 † (0.367)
Midwest	1.33 (0.274)	1.32 (0.274)
South	1.22 (0.232)	1.23 (0.236)
Number of Active Gangs	1.01 *** (0.002)	1.01 *** (0.002)
Number of Active Gang Members	0.999 ** (0.00003)	0.999 ** (0.00003)
Number of Years there has been a Gang Problem	1.03 *** (0.006)	1.02 *** (0.006)
Jurisdiction Population	1 *** (5.14)	1 *** (5.19)
Prior Level of Offending	1 (0.002)	0.999 (0.002)
Subsequent Level of Offending	1.01 *** (0.003)	1.01 *** (0.003)
Gang Unit or Officer	0.716 (0.149)	0.7504 (0.157)

*** $p < 0.001$; ** $p < 0.01$; * $p < 0.05$; † $p < 0.10$.

The results in Model 2 do not support the second hypothesis. The relationship between police reporting that gang migrants from outside United States significantly influence gang-related violence and gang-related homicides is negative, although it is not significant. Additional results reveal a significant and positive relationship between the number of active gangs and gang-related homicides, and a significant and negative association when comparing the number of active gang members and gang-related homicides. Moreover, the number of years there has been a gang problem, jurisdiction population, and increased likelihood of offending upon gang joining were all found to significantly increase the probability of gang-related homicide.

The results in Table 4 include Model 3, which consists of the percentage of gang migrants as the independent variable, and Model 4, which is the full model with percentage of gang migrants, police reporting of gang migrants from inside the U.S., and police reporting of gang migrants from outside the U.S. all significantly influencing gang-related violence.

Table 4. Percentage Gang Migrants and Gang-Related Homicides (n = 781).

Independent Variables	Model 3 I.R.R. (S.E.)	Model 4 I.R.R. (S.E.)
Percentage Gang Migrants	0.767 ** (0.069)	0.805 * (0.077)
Gang Migrants From U.S.	-	0.795 (0.139)
Gang Migrants from Outside of U.S.	-	0.861 (0.189)
Northeast	1.52 † (0.361)	1.49 † (0.353)
Midwest	1.35 (0.278)	1.32 (0.273)
South	1.204 (0.229)	1.17 (0.224)
Number of Active Gangs	1.01 *** (0.002)	1.01 *** (0.002)
Number of Active Gang Members	0.999 * (0.00003)	0.999 * (0.00003)
Number of Years there has been a Gang Problem	1.02 *** (0.006)	1.02 *** (0.006)
Jurisdiction Population	1 *** (5.32)	1 *** (5.33)
Prior Level of Offending	1 (0.002)	1 (0.002)
Subsequent Level of Offending	1.01 *** (0.003)	1.01 *** (0.003)
Gang Unit or Officer	0.747 (0.157)	0.727 (0.154)

*** $p < 0.001$; ** $p < 0.01$; * $p < 0.05$; † $p < 0.10$.

The results in Model 3 show support for the third hypothesis. There is a significant and negative association between the percentage of gang migrants in a jurisdiction and gang-related homicides. Additional findings reveal that the number of years there has been a gang problem, jurisdiction population, and increased likelihood of offending upon gang joining were all significant and positively associated with the likelihood of gang-related homicide. Furthermore, there is a significant and positive association between the number of active gangs and gang-related homicides, and a significant and negative association between the number of active gang members and gang-related homicides.

While the results in Model 4 show support for the third hypothesis, they do not support either the first or second hypotheses. There is a significant and negative association between the percentage of gang migrants in a jurisdiction and gang-related homicides. There is a negative association between police reporting that gang migrants within the U.S. influence gang-related violence and gang-related homicides, although it is not significant. The relationship between police reporting that gang migrants from outside the U.S. significantly influences gang-related violence and gang-related homicides is negative, although thus is not significant either. Additional findings reveal that the number of years there has been a gang problem, jurisdiction population, and increased likelihood of offending upon gang joining were all found to significantly increase the probability of gang-related homicides.

Moreover, there is a significant and positive relationship between the number of active gangs and gang-related homicides, and a significant and negative association when comparing the number of active gang members and gang-related homicides.

6. Summary of Findings and Discussion

Although Model 1 supported the first hypothesis, the full model (Model 4) did not show significant support for or against hypothesis one or two. Both Models 3 and 4 showed significant support for the third hypothesis, demonstrating that there is a significant and negative association between the percentage of gang members that are gang migrants in a community and the probability of gang-related homicides. The results suggest that gang migrants may aid in reducing the likelihood of serious crimes such as homicide. This is consistent with other research which has found that immigrants coming into a community can help to revitalize an area by strengthening social ties and support with one another, arguably reducing the likelihood of crime [11]. These findings are consistent with work examining gang migrants within the U.S. For example, Maxson (1997) found that although at times gang members may move for illicit reasons, most of the time they move for family-related or other social reasons. This suggests that they are not migrating in order to contribute to serious gang violence and homicide in the community.

Policy Implications

The results of this study highlight the need for community collaboration. Given that the presence of gang migrants significantly reduces the likelihood of gang-related homicides, communities should arguably be working to embrace and integrate these individuals into the area with the goal of reducing gang joining and other gang-related crimes. In areas where police may perceive and/or observe that gang migrants from within or outside the U.S. significantly contribute to gang-related violence, it is important to acknowledge that this does not necessarily result in an increase in the likelihood of gang-related homicides. Community education and exposure to gang migrant behavior could potentially bring perceptions in line with reality and help to reduce the likelihood of gang-related homicides as well as serious gang violence. It is important to adopt practices to aid in changing community perceptions of gang migrants. Therefore, it is essential to develop and utilize intervention methods that are culturally relevant [69]. This includes implementing methods that are family focused, adjusting perspectives, and providing resources for support.

The results highlight the need for community collaborative approaches to improve comprehension of gang migrant behavior. Specifically, if the presence of gang migrants significantly reduces the likelihood of gang-related homicides in a community, it is essential to understand why members are getting involved in gangs and the illegal behaviors they are engaging in. This could potentially be accomplished through community policing. Implementing community partnerships and collaborations that focus on communication, education, and the identification of the issues within specific areas will aid in improving community and police perceptions of gang migrants. By understanding their behaviors, the community can help address the needs of individuals who have recently relocated to their area, which may ultimately reduce the likelihood of other gang-related crimes as well.

Regional variation exists in gang member identification methods used by law enforcement in the United States [68]. More specifically, the use of gang signs and symbols to identify gang members is common [70]. Given that the presence of gang migrants decreases the likelihood of gang-related homicides, law enforcement may want to incorporate community collaboration into their gang member identification practices and protocols. Specifically, before officially identifying individuals as criminal gang members officers could communicate with members of the community to determine individual identity and status. This would strengthen overall community cohesion and potentially reduce both gang involvement among migrants and gang crime in general.

One of the biggest obstacles to this line of research is adjusting and improving both community and police perceptions of gang migrants. Community center or service projects may help with this. Bringing the community together for various social and/or service gatherings to improve an area, such as cleanup, can arguably help to change perceptions [71,72]. Research shows that individuals may join gangs due to feeling marginalized [73]. Youth born in the United States who experienced discrimination-related stress have a higher probability of gang involvement [74]. Causes of gang joining may vary for Latinos born in the U.S. compared to Latinos born elsewhere; this is because stress due to discrimination or adaptation is not a predictor of gang membership for immigrant youth, with economic inequality rather being reported as a major reason for gang joining. Based on the results of the current study, gang migrants do not relocate to become involved in serious violence, and preventing social and economic marginalization may aid in better relationships overall and potentially reduce the likelihood of migrants joining gangs as well as other gang-related crime.

7. Limitations and Conclusions

The data available on this topic are limited for a variety of reasons. This study is unable to establish causation. The data used were taken from the most recent NYGS and are cross-sectional. Thus, various control variables were utilized in a multivariate analytic approach in order to reduce the amount of spuriousness and to strengthen the findings. Although this is the most current available national data in the United States relating to the perspectives of law enforcement, future work will need to be conducted utilizing more current data in order to support the current findings. Furthermore, the percentage of gang migrants and of gang migrants influencing gang-related violence were determined through the perceptions of law enforcement. There are various limitations to using law enforcement perceptions to examine gang migrants, gang violence, and homicide. Law enforcement perspectives do not necessarily represent official crime data in a community, and rather represent the subjective opinions of law enforcement [75]; gang and member representations in the media may influence officer perspectives and result in implicit bias [76]. Future research will need to examine this issue from different community perspectives to better comprehend the relationship between gang migrants and gang related homicides and other crimes. Furthermore, it would be beneficial for future research to examine the relationship between gang migrants from both inside and outside of the United States and crime more generally.

In summation, the results of this study are consistent with past research examining immigration and crime. With a focus on gang migrants, this research contributes to the current literature by revealing that gang migrants reduce the likelihood of gang-related homicides in a jurisdiction. Given that gangs and gang members tend to be more likely to participate in crimes, including serious violence, compared to non-gang individuals, this work adds to the complexity of scholarship on gangs and gang involvement. Research has consistently argued for the need to have specialized gang policies and programs [77]. The current findings support this argument and suggest that focusing on collaboration between community groups and law enforcement will contribute to overall understanding of gang involvement, reduce the likelihood of serious gang violence, and improve relationships among newly-arrived and longtime members of the community.

Funding: This research received no external funding.

Institutional Review Board Statement: Ethical review and approval were not required for this study, due to the data being publicly available with no individual identifiers.

Informed Consent Statement: The current study is secondary data analysis, but informed consent was obtained when the data was originally collected.

Data Availability Statement: Data for the National Youth Gang Survey can be accessed through the Inter-university Consortium for Political and Social Research (icpsr.umich.edu).

Conflicts of Interest: The authors declare no conflict of interest.

Notes

[1] Although "gang migrants" frequently refers to gang members moving from one jurisdiction to another within the same country, it can refer to gang members moving from one country to another as well; see van Gemert et al., 2008.

[2] Outliers dropped.

References

1. Decker, S.H.; Melde, C.; Pyrooz, D.C. What do we know about gangs and gang members and where do we go from here? *Justice Q.* **2013**, *30*, 369–402. [CrossRef]
2. Adams, J.J.; Pizarro, J.M. Patterns of specialization and escalation in the criminal careers of gang and non-gang homicide offenders. *Crim. Justice Behav.* **2014**, *41*, 237–255. [CrossRef]
3. Papachristos, A.V. Murder by structure: Dominance relations and the social structure of gang homicide. *Am. J. Sociol.* **2009**, *115*, 74–128. [CrossRef] [PubMed]
4. Sanchez, J.A.; Decker, S.H.; Pyrooz, D.C. Gang homicide: The road so far and a map for the future. *Homicide Stud.* **2021**, *26*, 68–90. [CrossRef]
5. Maxson, C.L. *Gang Members on the Move*; Office of Juvenile Justice and Delinquency Prevention: Washington, DC, USA, 1997.
6. Hagedorn, J.M.; Macon, P. *People and Folks. Gangs, Crime and the Underclass in a Rustbelt City*; Lake View Press: Chicago, IL, USA, 1988.
7. Skolnick, J.H.; Correl, T.; Navaro, E.; Rabb, R. *The Social Structure of Street Drug Dealing*; BCS Forum, Office of Attorney General: Sacramento, CA, USA; p. 1988.
8. Waldorf, D. When the Crips invaded San Francisco: Gang migration. *J. Gang Res.* **1993**, *1*, 11–16.
9. Zevitz, R.G.; Takata, S.R. Metropolitan gang influence and the emergence of group delinquency in a regional community. *J. Crim. Justice* **1992**, *20*, 93–106. [CrossRef]
10. Emerick, N.A.; Curry, T.R.; Collins, T.W.; Fernando Rodriguez, S. Homicide and social disorganization on the border: Implications for Latino and immigrant populations. *Soc. Sci. Q.* **2014**, *95*, 360–379. [CrossRef]
11. Chouhy, C.; Madero-Hernandez, A. "Murderers, Rapists, and Bad Hombres": Deconstructing the Immigration-Crime Myths. *Vict. Offenders* **2019**, *14*, 1010–1039. [CrossRef]
12. Vargas, R.; Scrivener, L. Why Latino youth (don't) call police. *Race Justice* **2021**, *11*, 47–64. [CrossRef]
13. Correia, M.E. Determinants of attitudes toward police of Latino immigrants and non-immigrants. *J. Crim. Justice* **2010**, *38*, 99–107. [CrossRef]
14. Durán, R.J. *The Gang Paradox: Inequalities and Miracles on the US-Mexico border*; Columbia University Press: New York, NY, USA, 2018.
15. Decker, S.H. Collective and normative features of gang violence. *Justice Q.* **1996**, *13*, 243–264. [CrossRef]
16. Thornberry, T.P.; Krohn, M.D.; Lizotte, A.J.; Smith, C.A.; Tobin, K. *Gangs and Delinquency in Developmental Perspective*; Cambridge University Press: Cambridge, UK, 2003.
17. Pyrooz, D.C.; Turanovic, J.J.; Decker, S.H.; Wu, J. Taking stock of the relationship between gang membership and offending: A meta-analysis. *Crim. Justice Behav.* **2016**, *43*, 365–397. [CrossRef]
18. Moore, J.W.; Garcia, R.; Moore, J.W.; Garcia, C. *Homeboys: Gangs, Drugs, and Prison in the Barrios of Los Angeles*; Temple University Press: Philadelphia, PA, USA, 1978.
19. Scott, D. A comparison of gang-and non-gang-related violent incidents from the incarcerated youth perspective. *Deviant Behav.* **2018**, *39*, 1336–1356. [CrossRef]
20. Adamson, C. Defensive localism in white and black: A comparative history of European-American and African-American youth gangs. *Ethn. Racial Stud.* **2000**, *23*, 272–298. [CrossRef]
21. Alonso, A.A. Racialized identitites and the formation of black gangs in Los Angeles. *Urban Geogr.* **2004**, *25*, 658–674. [CrossRef]

22. Decker, S.H.; Van Gemert, F.; Pyrooz, D.C. Gangs, migration, and crime: The changing landscape in Europe and the USA. *J. Int. Migr. Integr./Rev. L'integration La Migr. Int.* **2009**, *10*, 393–408. [CrossRef]
23. Hagedorn, J.M. Race not space: A revisionist history of gangs in Chicago. *J. Afr. Am. Hist.* **2006**, *91*, 194–208. [CrossRef]
24. Klein, M.W. *The American Street Gang: Its Nature, Prevalence, and Control*; Oxford University Press: Oxford, UK, 1997.
25. Decker, S.H.; Curry, G.D. Gangs, gang homicides, and gang loyalty: Organized crimes or disorganized criminals. *J. Crim. Justice* **2002**, *30*, 343–352. [CrossRef]
26. Tita, G.; Abrahamse, A. Gang Homicide in LA, 1981–2001. At the Local Level: Perspectives on Violence Prevention. In *At the Local Level: Perspectives on Violence Prevention*; California Attorney General's Office: San Francisco, CA, USA, 2004; 3, pp. 1–20.
27. Howell, J.C. Youth gang homicides: A literature review. *Crime Delinq.* **1999**, *45*, 208–241. [CrossRef]
28. Maxson, C.L. Gang homicide: A review and extension of the literature. In *Homicide: A Sourcebook of Social Research*; Sage Publications: Thousand Oaks, CA, USA, 1999; pp. 239–254.
29. Maxson, C.L.; Curry, G.D.; Howell, J.C. Youth gang homicides in the United States in the 1990s. In *Responding to Gangs: Evaluation and Research*; U.S. Department of Justice, Office of Justice Programs, National Institute of Justice: Washington, DC, USA, 2002; pp. 107–137.
30. Valasik, M.; Reid, S.E. East Side Story: Disaggregating Gang Homicides in East Los Angeles. *Soc. Sci.* **2021**, *10*, 48. [CrossRef]
31. Cohen, J.; Tita, G. Diffusion in homicide: Exploring a general method for detecting spatial diffusion processes. *J. Quant. Criminol.* **1999**, *15*, 451–493. [CrossRef]
32. Miller, J.; Decker, S.H. Young women and gang violence: Gender, street offending, and violent victimization in gangs. *Justice Q.* **2001**, *18*, 115–140. [CrossRef]
33. Rosenfeld, R.; Bray, T.M.; Egley, A. Facilitating violence: A comparison of gang-motivated, gang-affiliated, and nongang youth homicides. *J. Quant. Criminol.* **1999**, *15*, 495–516. [CrossRef]
34. Maxson, C.L.; Gordon, M.A.; Klein, M.W. Differences between gang and nongang homicides. *Criminology* **1985**, *23*, 209–222. [CrossRef]
35. Urbanik, M.M.; Roks, R.A. Making sense of murder: The reality versus the realness of gang homicides in two contexts. *Soc. Sci.* **2021**, *10*, 17. [CrossRef]
36. Stretesky, P.B.; Pogrebin, M.R. Gang-related gun violence: Socialization, identity, and self. *J. Contemp. Ethnogr.* **2007**, *36*, 85–114. [CrossRef]
37. Brotherton, D. *Youth Street Gangs: A Critical Appraisal*; Routledge: London, UK, 2015.
38. Pyrooz, D.C. Structural covariates of gang homicide in large US cities. *J. Res. Crime Delinq.* **2012**, *49*, 489–518. [CrossRef]
39. Bonfante, J. Entrepreneurs of Crack. Available online: http://content.time.com/time/subscriber/article/0,33009,982588,00.html (accessed on 14 December 2021).
40. Genelin, M.; Coplen, B. Los Angeles Street Gangs: Report and Recommendations of the County-Wide Criminal Justice Coordination Committee Interagency Gang Task Force, March 1989. Los Angeles: Interagency Gang Task Force. 1989. Available online: https://www.ojp.gov/ncjrs/virtual-library/abstracts/california-council-criminal-justice-state-task-force-gangs-and (accessed on 21 June 2021).
41. National Drug Intelligence Center. *Blood and Crips Gang Survey Report*; National Drug Intelligence Center: Johnstown, PA, USA, 1994.
42. National Drug Intelligence Center. *National Street Gang Survey Report*; National Drug Intelligence Center: Johnstown, PA, USA, 1996.
43. Egley, A.; Howell, C. *Highlights of the 2010 National Youth Gang Survey*; US Department of Justice Office of Juvenile Justice and Delinquency Prevention: Washington, DC, USA, 2012.
44. Howell, J.C.; Griffiths, E. *Gangs in America's Communities*; Sage Publications: Thousand Oaks, CA, USA, 2018.
45. Van Gemert, F.; Decker, S. Migrant Groups and Gang Activity: A Contrast between Europe and the USA (From Street Gangs, Migration and Ethnicity). In *Street Gangs, Migration and Ethnicity*; van Gemert, F., Peterson, D., Lien, I.-L., Eds.; Willan Publishing: Milton, UK, 2008; pp. 15–30.
46. Kelly, K.; Caputo, T. The linkages between street gangs and organized crime: The Canadian experience. *J. Gang Res.* **2005**, *13*, 17–31.
47. Maxson, C.L. Investigating gang migration: Contextual issues. *Gang J.* **1993**, *1*, 1–8.
48. McGuire, C. Washington Office on Latin America January, 2007 Central American Youth Gangs in the Washington DC Area. 2006. Available online: https://www.wola.org/analysis/youth-gangs-in-central-america/ (accessed on 11 November 2021).
49. Lee, E. *At America's Gates: Chinese Immigration during the Exclusion Era, 1882–1943*; University of North Carolina Press: Chapel Hill, NC, USA, 2003.
50. Lee, M.T.; Martinez, R.; Rosenfeld, R. Does immigration increase homicide? Negative evidence from three border cities. *Sociol. Q.* **2001**, *42*, 559–580. [CrossRef]
51. Martinez, R., Jr.; Rosenfeld, R.; Mares, D. Social disorganization, drug market activity, and neighborhood violent crime. *Urban Aff. Rev.* **2008**, *43*, 846–874. [CrossRef] [PubMed]
52. Martinez, R., Jr.; Stowell, J.I.; Lee, M.T. Immigration and crime in an era of transformation: A longitudinal analysis of homicides in San Diego neighborhoods, 1980–2000. *Criminology* **2010**, *48*, 797–829. [CrossRef]

53. Reid, L.W.; Weiss, H.E.; Adelman, R.M.; Jaret, C. The immigration–crime relationship: Evidence across US metropolitan areas. *Soc. Sci. Res.* **2005**, *34*, 757–780. [CrossRef]
54. Stowell, J.I.; Messner, S.F.; McGeever, K.F.; Raffalovich, L.E. Immigration and the recent violent crime drop in the United States: A pooled, cross-sectional time-series analysis of metropolitan areas. *Criminology* **2009**, *47*, 889–928. [CrossRef]
55. Wadsworth, T. Is immigration responsible for the crime drop? An assessment of the influence of immigration on changes in violent crime between 1990 and 2000. *Soc. Sci. Q.* **2010**, *91*, 531–553. [CrossRef]
56. Brown, B.; Benedict, W.R. Bullets, blades, and being afraid in Hispanic high schools: An exploratory study of the presence of weapons and fear of weapon-associated victimization among high school students in a border town. *Crime Delinq.* **2004**, *50*, 372–394. [CrossRef]
57. Martinez, R., Jr. *Latino Homicide: Immigration, Violence, and Community*; Routledge: London, UK, 2014.
58. Kubrin, C.E.; Ousey, G.C. Immigration and Homicide in Urban America: What's the Connection? In *Immigration, Crime and Justice*; Emerald Group Publishing Limited: Bingley, UK, 2009.
59. Menjívar, C.; Bejarano, C. Latino immigrants' perceptions of crime and police authorities in the United States: A case study from the Phoenix metropolitan area. *Ethn. Racial Stud.* **2004**, *27*, 120–148. [CrossRef]
60. Tapia, M. Gangs in the El Paso-Juárez borderland: The role of history and geography in shaping criminal subcultures. *Trends Organ. Crime* **2020**, *23*, 367–384. [CrossRef]
61. Barak, M.P.; León, K.S.; Maguire, E.R. Conceptual and empirical obstacles in defining MS-13: Law-enforcement perspectives. *Criminol. Public Policy* **2020**, *19*, 563–589. [CrossRef]
62. Esbensen, F.A.; Carson, D.C. Who are the gangsters? An examination of the age, race/ethnicity, sex, and immigration status of self-reported gang members in a seven-city study of American youth. *J. Contemp. Crim. Justice* **2012**, *28*, 465–481. [CrossRef]
63. Valdez, A.; Cepeda, A.; Kaplan, C. Homicidal events among Mexican American street gangs: A situational analysis. *Homicide Stud.* **2009**, *13*, 288–306. [CrossRef] [PubMed]
64. Hollis, M.E. The impact of population and economic decline: Examining socio-demographic correlates of homicide in Detroit. *Crime Prev. Community Saf.* **2018**, *20*, 84–98. [CrossRef]
65. Decker, S.H.; Pyrooz, D.C. On the validity and reliability of gang homicide: A comparison of disparate sources. *Homicide Stud.* **2010**, *14*, 359–376. [CrossRef]
66. Rubin, D.B. *Multiple Imputation for Nonresponse in Surveys*; Wiley: New York, NY, USA, 1987.
67. Schafer, J.L. *Analysis of Incomplete Multivariate Data*; Chapman & Hall/CRC: Boca Raton, FL, USA, 1997.
68. Scott, D. Regional differences in gang member identification methods among law enforcement jurisdictions in the United States. *Polic. Int. J.* **2020**, *43*, 723–740. [CrossRef]
69. Dominguez, J.; Puls, L. The Impact of Culturally Relevant Programs: Research Snapshot. 2020. Available online: https://victimresearch.org/library/culturally-relevant-programs/ (accessed on 9 January 2022).
70. Densley, J.A.; Pyrooz, D.C. The matrix in context: Taking stock of police gang databases in London and beyond. *Youth Justice* **2020**, *20*, 11–30. [CrossRef]
71. Baillie, L.; Bromley, B.; Walker, M.; Jones, R.; Mhlanga, F. Implementing service improvement projects within pre-registration nursing education: A multi-method case study evaluation. *Nurse Educ. Pract.* **2014**, *14*, 62–68. [CrossRef] [PubMed]
72. Waterman, A.S. An overview of service-learning and the role of research and evaluation in service-learning programs. In *Service-Learning*; Routledge: London, UK, 2014; pp. 15–26.
73. Vigil, J.D.; Yun, S.C. A cross-cultural framework for understanding gangs: Multiple marginality and Los Angeles. *Gangs Am.* **2002**, *3*, 161–174.
74. Barrett, A.N.; Kuperminc, G.P.; Lewis, K.M. Acculturative stress and gang involvement among Latinos: US-born versus immigrant youth. *Hisp. J. Behav. Sci.* **2013**, *35*, 370–389. [CrossRef]
75. Carson, D.; Hipple, N.K. Comparing violent and non-violent gang incidents: An exploration of gang-related police incident reports. *Soc. Sci.* **2020**, *9*, 199. [CrossRef]
76. Esbensen, F.A.; Tusinski, K.E. Youth gangs in the print media. *J. Crim. Justice Pop. Cult.* **2007**, *14*, 21–38.
77. Valasik, M.; Reid, S.E. Taking stock of gang violence: An overview of the literature. In *Handbook of Interpersonal Violence across the Lifespan*; Springer: New York, NY, USA, 2019; pp. 1–21.

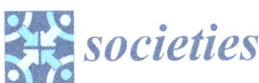

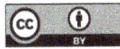

Article

Finding a Suitable Object for Intervention: On Community-Based Violence Prevention in Sweden

Kristina Alstam [1,*] **and Torbjörn Forkby** [2]

1   Department of Social Work, University of Gothenburg, 405 30 Gothenburg, Sweden
2   Department of Social Work, Linnaeus University, 351 95 Växjö, Sweden; torbjorn.forkby@lnu.se
*   Correspondence: kristina.alstam@socwork.gu.se

Abstract: In Sweden, local municipalities, working in collaboration with the police, are assigned an important role in community-based crime prevention and the promotion of safer neighbourhoods/cities. The strategies adopted are supposed to be informed by the policies of national advisory bodies, which emphasize surveying the current situation, problem analyses, systematic planning of interventions and evaluation of efforts. This paper reports on a three-year research project that studied local crime prevention/safer community practices in four so-called 'particularly vulnerable areas' (PVAs) using meeting observations and stakeholder interviews. The analysis shows that when constructing intervention strategies, the actors involved had to navigate between different organizational logics and found it difficult to demarcate a suitable object for joint efforts. When they were able to find an object to be targeted, such as youth at risk of drug abuse or low-level criminality, they could rely on a collective mindset, but they struggled in situations where a joint effort was not possible, such as when dealing with the risk of aggravated violence or when the operations got close to more organized crime—both elements that form part of the definition of PVAs. This failure may partly be explained by competing logics dominated by idiosyncratic action in line with bureaucratic rules and routines. This finding raises questions about a putative but non-articulated limit to crime prevention and whether a predetermined approach aligns with the prescribed sequence of survey, analysis, intervention planning and evaluation when faced with more brutish violence.

Keywords: collaborative crime prevention; organizational logics; intervention; violence; particularly vulnerable areas

Citation: Alstam, K.; Forkby, T. Finding a Suitable Object for Intervention: On Community-Based Violence Prevention in Sweden. *Societies* **2022**, *12*, 75. https://doi.org/10.3390/soc12030075

Academic Editors: Jaimee Mallion and Erika Gebo

Received: 4 March 2022
Accepted: 25 April 2022
Published: 29 April 2022

Publisher's Note: MDPI stays neutral with regard to jurisdictional claims in published maps and institutional affiliations.

1. Introduction

In recent years, Sweden has focused increasingly on gang-related criminality and how it is related to the situation in more marginalized neighbourhoods. The policy response has generally prioritized repressive interventions such as allocating more resources to the police, tapping phone calls and messages, assigning longer sentences for gang-related crimes, and reducing the 'youth reduction' that reduces imprisonment time for younger persons. Concerns have also been raised about local authorities' competence and the prioritization of preventive measures, not least the readiness of municipal organizations and police for coordinated strategies and operations [1,2].

The most influential document framing political discussion and media coverage was the first *NOA Report* presented in 2015 by the national police. It introduced the concept of 'vulnerable areas' (in later reports also referred to as 'areas of risk', and 'particularly vulnerable areas'), thus inventing a term that embraced drug sales, uprisings against the police, violent crime, undue influence on law enforcement agencies, religious extremism and so-called 'parallel societies'. The solutions suggested spreading the responsibility for action across a wide partnership of local authorities and services such as social services, local schools, leisure administration, local churches and health centres, which were to work hand in hand with the police. The intensification of voices calling for increased collaboration among stakeholders and a more systematic and knowledge-based approach have led to a legislative bill that is to be enacted in 2023. The bill will make it compulsory for municipalities to develop strategies for and engage in crime prevention collaboration [3] (p. 49).

The need to upgrade locally situated crime prevention has a long history. The world's first crime prevention council was launched in 1974 to inform policymaking by analysing crime fluctuations in order to provide guidance on crime prevention strategies [4]. The national crime prevention programme *Everybody's Responsibility* [1] was released in 1997, to be replaced by *Together Against Crime* [2] in 2017. Both policy documents emphasized the need for collaboration between authorities to reduce crime, with the latter document phrasing this more strongly. At present there is a nationwide organizational structure including the national advisory body, county level coordinators, local crime prevention councils at the strategic municipal level, and local groups responsible for the operative work at the district level.

The collaborative structures at the strategic and operative level in the municipalities have a history that can be traced back several decades in Swedish crime prevention history. An operative level involving social services, municipal police, district schools and youth centres has been recommended since the beginning of the 1970s [5]. These groups have regular meetings where they address issues relating to potentially vulnerable young people at risk of involvement in drug use, criminality or recruitment by known criminals. However, although Swedish initiatives for local crime prevention were implemented several years ago, they have been studied only to a moderate degree (see however [6–8]).

This paper stems from a three-year long research project started in 2019 that investigated collaborative crime prevention strategies and settings in four of Sweden's particularly vulnerable areas (PVAs), or 'superdiverse' neighbourhoods [9]. The aim was to identify the logics that regulate local crime prevention practices and assess whether the policy recommendation of a systematic problem-solving process is applicable, and if not, why not.

Crime prevention is understood here as a broad term including intentional measures and circumstances that decrease the probability of criminality or reduce the harm from crime [10]. It thus includes interventions both before and after a criminal act has occurred. In the latter case, it might involve taking action to counter the risk of aggravated circles of violence and counter attacks, as well as trying to cushion the effects of stress and protect safety at the community level after an incident. This definition fits well with the assignment given to the crime prevention settings that are the focus of the study, namely, that they are to address both the symptoms and the mechanisms behind the problematic aspects of PVAs. However, given the fact that the collaborative prevention groups traditionally have addressed delinquent youth groups and low-level crimes, what happens when they are confronted by heavy criminality and intertwined links between organized criminality and rowdy behaviour among youth? This paper aims to probe into the manner in which the prescribed logics for interventions work when the collaborative preventive settings face situations associated with organised crime and/or a risk of aggravated violence.

2. Collaborative and Systematic Crime Prevention

Nordic crime prevention has traditionally aimed at a combination of situational prevention and social welfare policies [11]. The chief institutional actor in the field of crime prevention in Sweden is the Council for Crime Prevention (CCP), operating under the Ministry of Justice. The CCP can be described as an institute mainly initiating and circulating research in the domain, including hands-on methodological knowledge about crime prevention [8]. The CCP's methodological guidance lays out a prescribed sequence of professional actions that need to be carried out if crime prevention is to reach its goals. The work is to be conducted in a 'systematized' fashion and is ordained to include the following steps: (1) surveying the problem, (2) analysing the problem, (3) prioritizing the correct measures, (4) implementing the measures and, lastly, (5) evaluating the results. To produce a broad understanding of a particular problem, the participating actors are supposed to merge their perceptions into one that encapsulates the complexity of the phenomenon. Although the details of this systematic strategy were not top of mind for the various leaders involved in the collaborative settings we studied, they were all familiar with the general idea of the different phases and what type of work they involved.

Some attempts to work according to the CCP recommendations have been evaluated, such as the method known as *Effective Collaboration for Increased Security* (EST). The professionals expressed a need for an enhanced structure and organization, and noted that working according to EST seemed more flexible and better theoretically supported. The professionals involved expressed a perception of more systematized and structured crime preventive work [7].

3. Previous Research

Collaborative efforts clearly have a long history in Swedish crime prevention policy, but their present ideological and methodological encapsulation is indebted to the multi-agency/partnership approaches articulated by New Labour during the mid 1990s. The intention to be both 'tough on crime, and tough on its causes' was translated into managerial efficiency, long-term agreements between stakeholders, and the design of tailor-made local strategies to promote safety and prevent crime [12–14]. While the partnership model has been a success with respect to the international exchange of policy initiatives, it still has a lot to prove in terms of its capacity to sustain what is envisioned [15].

Crime prevention programmes, and especially the practice of prevention, are seldom evidence-based [16] or adapted to tackle different target groups, places and type of crimes [17]. The potential effects of a programme will depend upon what is supposed to be changed, e.g., opportunities for crime, the mechanisms that fuel individual motivation, or group dynamics between rowdy youth. This variability places high demands on a preventionist's competence [18]. The idea that crime prevention should rely on established models or assigned methods [7] becomes problematic when confronted by new and evolving situations. The requirement to integrate the ideas of different parties when assessing strategies can obstruct a plan to find more well-documented methods.

Even if the intention in the partnership policy is to focus on the broader structure, signalled by 'safer city' approaches, actual practice often focuses more narrowly on individuals [13], and thus transfers responsibility for safety lower in the hierarchy [19]. However, involving residents has not been as easy as is assumed in the policy documents [20–22]. A key to forming a successful partnership seems to be including local coordinators and providing training and assessable guidance in crime prevention [23,24], provided that their role is given the required mandate for the assignment [6,25]. As Harkin [26] argues, the question is perhaps not whether partnership works or not, but when and what issues are suitable for the partners. The police may often get more out of a partnership than the other parties [27].

In terms of crime prevention efficiency, there is much room for improvement, not least regarding the methods used and the collaboration, as well as in terms of partnering with citizens [15,28–30].

A substantial part of the crime prevention literature has been concerned with place-based prevention and hot-spots policing, showing generally small or moderate positive effects (e.g., [31–35]). However, the partnerships also involve social prevention, which translates into more ambiguous processes, even more so when the issue is to prevent violence. Programmes designed to prevent violence at a community level are not easily evaluated as they are geared toward impacting both protective and risk factors, which makes it difficult to ascertain their success [36]. Two well-known exceptions that target gang-related violence and include the community level are the Chicago Ceasefire programme [37] and Focused Deterrence [38]. The latter has begun to be implemented in Sweden [39].

From their experience supporting crime prevention in deprived neighbourhoods in Tulsa, OK, USA, Corsaro and Engel [40] propose a number of key factors for effective partnerships: (a) mobilizing resources widely among public institutions, community groups, business representatives, etc.; (b) giving time to build trust and form long-term commitment; (c) employing a structured work process (surveying, planning and executing interventions) supplied with well-founded feedback; (d) including a varied tool box of interventions serving to facilitate local norm building, social support and local capacity; (e) working in alliance between (embedded) researchers and practitioners (see [41]). Even if these factors are familiar to partnerships internationally, British experiences show that variations in overall aims decide the balance between the components [27]; furthermore, the implementation in Germany was uneven and not supported by evidence and had hard time integrating citizen perspectives [42], while the influence in Spain was hampered from the lack of a supporting national framework [43], and the reduction in crime, somewhat paradoxically, resulted in a decreased interest in safer city/partnership approaches [44].

4. The Study: Data Collection and Analysis

The data for this paper were collected during a three-year research project starting in 2019 [3]. The focus was on the practices employed in crime prevention, how safety is understood and facilitated, and what capacity the collaborative operations had when responding to the situation in four PVAs. Data from two of the PVAs were chosen for deeper analysis, while data from the other two were used to inform and check this analysis. We observed and took fieldnotes of 34 collaborative meetings at the operative and strategic levels and interviewed 29 stakeholders from the top municipal level and managerial level down to the operative level for the two PVAs chosen. Five days of shadowing local coordinators are also included in the data.

The research process was discussed within the research group throughout the project. A research handbook for the project was worked out before the data were collected, describing how to proceed with the different methods to be used.

The observations were guided by a structured scheme including background data for meetings, actual participants and the issues brought up. We also concentrated on the dynamics within the meetings, such as whether questions were posed, when information was given, whether different opinions were articulated and how potential conflicts were handled. Fieldnotes were taken to support the observation sheet and provide emerging ideas for the analysis.

The interviews were semi-structured to allow interviewees to talk freely and share their views on preventive collaboration and to obtain information on each interviewee's own organization's task and responsibilities.

The analysis contained both quantitative observations of the meetings and thematic qualitative analyses of processes during the meetings. The overarching findings of the project, partly presented in this paper, are anchored in the four case study reports and their associated data. However, the results include a deeper analysis of the way challenges to crime prevention practices have resulted in a concentration on critical incidents, together with obstacles faced and strategies adopted. The empirical extracts chosen for analysis were selected on the basis of their exposing recurrent features of the meetings observed.

5. Projected Knowledge

The formal task for the crime prevention councils is to assess present situations, make assumptions about potential future developments and identify what actions should be undertaken to improve the odds for preferred outcomes. The resources available for this process are mainly the actors' knowledge of the local community, their theoretical and practical experience, and the organizational resources they can allocate to making things happen. All of this is framed by what the organizations will allow, the dynamics within the prevention group, and what knowledge they collectively have at their disposal. From this viewpoint, the practice of prevention is a case of organizationally bounded knowledge use in which specific professionals plan to restrict or promote mechanisms that affect future events.

Lam [45] points out the 'interactive relationship between dominant knowledge types and organizational forms' (p. 487). Collaboration thus imposes a non-articulated demand that separate knowledge types and organizational forms coalesce. An important feature of collaborative practices is that they exhibit some characteristics of being organizations in themselves and simultaneously are betwixt and between organizations. This means that the actors have a double identity and divided loyalties and will have to negotiate the mandate to define which 'orders for action' will dominate the groups. These orders relate to the concept of institutional logics [46], meaning direction indicators coming from the particular organization's design and knowledge types, as well as its value system, chains of command and working practices.

A steering philosophy that would sit well with the policy ideal of a systematic but still innovative order of action would be to organise the work as a project flow guided by project management [47]. Assessment and decision-making would be guided by pre-structured instruments with theoretical underpinnings. A mandated coordinator would lead the process and a dedicated group would target the actual problem, drawing on available resources while relatively free from other obligations or administrative restrictions. Such a logic would take the best from a routine-based bureaucracy, meritocratic openness to dialogue and adhocratic readiness to act and use embodied knowledge in uncertain and unpredictable situations (see [48,49]).

When evaluating a situation and reaching a decision on how to act, the interplay of the organisational form and logic with different kinds of knowledge is a key feature. At an epistemological level, there is the issue of explicit and tacit knowledge to consider. Explicit knowledge is normally manifest and can be codified. It is easy to abstract, communicate and store without the participation of the knowing subject. Tacit knowledge is unarticulated, action-oriented and almost intuitive. It is less easy to communicate, understand or apply without guidance from a knowing subject. Transferring tacit knowledge takes close interaction and a shared understanding [45] (p. 490).

Explicit knowledge can be acquired by formal study, while tacit knowledge is generated through practical experience. Even the ways in which the two forms of knowledge can be aggregated differ. Explicit knowledge can be aggregated at a single site. It can be stockpiled and reached without assistance from the knowing subject. Tacit knowledge works the other way around: it is produced in a particular context and it is personal. To access it, one needs to cooperate in close involvement with the knowing subject [45] (p. 490).

There is also an ontological dimension of knowledge, configured as a matter of individual versus collective knowledge. The first is domain-specific, specialized and accumulated within a single person's body or brain, which makes it a case of bounded rationality [50]. Since it is autonomous and moves with the individual holding it, the accumulation of such knowledge is precarious [45] (p. 491). Collective knowledge, on the other hand, is held by an organization itself and deposited in its norms, routines and procedures. It is fertilized in communicative action among professionals, and comes to life *between*, rather than within, individuals [51].

All organizations normally manifest a mix of the knowledge forms. Lam [45] (p. 493) suggests the following model that brings together the epistemological and ontological forms to show their manifestations within an organizational framework, see Figure 1 below:

| | | Ontological dimension | |
		individual	collective
Epistemological dimension	explicit	*Embrained knowledge*	*Encoded knowledge*
	tacit	*Embodied knowledge*	*Embedded knowledge*

Figure 1. Logics for decision making in respect to different types of knowledge.

Embrained knowledge is the combination of individual and explicit knowledge. It is based on theories and depends on the individual's conceptual skills. Embodied knowledge (which is individual and tacit) is action oriented. It is a type of knowledge that requires practical experience. Encoded knowledge is a combination of collective and explicit knowledge forms and could be summarized as that which we label 'information'. It is codified and stored in written rules and procedures and it may predict patterns of behaviour and output in organizations. Lastly, embedded knowledge is a combination of the collective and tacit knowledge categories and can be understood as the tacit knowledge embedded in shared norms and organizational routines. This knowledge comes from a shared understanding and is relation-specific, contextual, organic and dynamic and applied in the absence of written rules.

The requirement to operate in the recommended systematic, phase-regulated fashion in an unstable environment while making assessments and reaching decisions in a collaborative setting in-between organizations places high demands on the competence of the actors involved. They must translate the meaning of regulations and routines from their mother organizations into a new context, and articulate which aspects of their embrained, encoded, embodied and embedded knowledge are applicable. This requires the group to evolve as a community of practice [52], constructing in negotiation both a mutual group identity and an amalgamated knowledge base.

6. Results

The results will be presented in terms of three themes that together show the prevention constellations' responses when confronted with complex situations of violence and crime. The first, *preventionist creaming*, refers to the tendency for crime prevention groups to work on the basis of previously established patterns and with the issues that are most accessible for them. The next theme, *pulling intertwined strings*, shows the difficulties of planning for action when a situation requires deep insider knowledge and different perspectives block resolution. Lastly, the theme *prevention as a double-edged sword* probes the question of strategic planning when it is very hard to envisage whether the consequence of taking action will exacerbate the situation rather than alleviate it.

6.1. Preventionist Creaming

A vital insight when seeking to understand collaborative crime preventive settings is that the work is often commonplace. Even when the professionals are dedicated to the severely marginalized communities described in political debates and the media as controlled by criminal elements, they are to a great extent occupied with teenagers found in the wrong places at the wrong time, neighbourhood beatings, shopkeepers selling illegal fireworks, or loitering with intent to commit theft. Even when confronted with more severe crimes, attention is often steered towards previously constructed knowledge bases and cases that are more easily demarcated. This can be seen as a practice of creaming, separating what could be intervention objects from the more complex issues in need of a structured analysis and plan of action. As a consequence, efforts often focus on situational measures such as lighting and camera surveillance, or on social measures such as intervening in conflicts or drug use among teenagers at the local high school [32].

The collaboration that does take place is invested in updating the collective awareness of the day-to-day fluctuations in the neighbourhood. This is often translated into a ritual of going around the meeting table as the participants (e.g., the police, social workers, school representatives, housing companies and youth workers) present concerns about what has been going on. There may be questions and discussion during this part of the meeting, but usually the focus is on sharing information rather than on more substantial analysis.

This lack of analysis has been observed as a general problem when evaluating crime prevention settings in Sweden [53]. There are a few (but not many) examples of more systematic analyses seeking to bring the parent organizations together under a broader umbrella of local crime prevention. However, this only seems to happen when there is a specific issue to be addressed and a specific setup of actors. The example below from case A, a PVA in a medium-size city (100,000 inhabitants) in Sweden, indicates that such an analysis is easier when it comes to more mundane aspects of keeping the environment nice and tidy.

> The foundation Safer Sweden was asked to perform a safety analysis in [case A] last autumn. And they produced a plan of action with concrete measures and later long-term goals. . . . And it is . . . It places the emphasis on the physical environment. That is, how to make changes in the physical environment to increase security and that stuff. But we try to . . . Now we talk to, well the housing companies in A, on getting a joint project to ensure that we have guaranteed . . . Yes, for example to pick up litter and manage walkways . . . You see, there are many things of that nature they pick up in analysis. (Security coordinator in A)

By contrast, observation of the work performed by the security coordinator in case B, situated in the suburbs of a large Swedish city (600,000 inhabitants), revealed that matters of a more trivial nature were addressed alongside issues relating to serious crime and violence.

During one and the same meeting with housing companies, security coordinators and caretakers, the group discussed (a) plans to tackle matters of parking surveillance and incorrect parking, and (b) a murder in a residential area close to B. In the meeting observed, the murder was dealt with only by giving sparse information and leaving the solution to the police, while the lion's share of the meeting was dedicated to parking matters. This is not surprising given that the required preliminary investigation secrecy prevents the police from providing information to the participants, and the fact that the police was not present at the meeting. It nevertheless shows that the dominance of the organizational logic [48] can be present simply through information. Perhaps the fact that the police were to address the matter, hampered all other initiatives from the group. Even though the murder could not be prevented any longer, the group could have considered the risk of revenge attacks and countering the spreading of rumours as part of a prevention strategy to counter violence in the community. However, the more easily demarcated subject for joint deliberations and interventions around parking concerns caught their attention.

It may be that the group lacked a collective knowledge base on how to act in the context of murder. By processing explicit and tacit knowledge, they had previously succeeded in forming alliances to deal with unruly teenagers, parking tickets and cartridges of laughing gas being found near the shopping mall. However, when confronted by the murder, they did not step up as preventionists, and seemed to be lacking 'adhocratic' motivation to reduce its harmful effects at the community level. This preventionist creaming, meaning a restriction of collective efforts into the perceived manageable in respect to organizational boundaries, knowledge base and previous practices, may also block attempts to find deeper causes of crime, something Gilling [13] has pointed out as a main shortcoming of these attempts. This, in turn, may relate to another finding in the study: the perception from the preventionists that they indeed possess knowledge about causes for crime, but lack the necessary mandate to address it.

6.2. Pulling Intertwined Strings

When it comes to violence prevention, it can be difficult to carve out a suitable object of intervention because of the complexity of a situation, even if the group has scope to act before (worse) violence occurs and is free from the influence of other organizations in the planning phase.

The meeting from which the following field notes stem was commissioned for the social services and the police in case B. The group met on a weekly basis to jointly address matters involving young offenders, specifically to prevent cycles of retaliation and progression to more serious criminal activities.

> Incident of a ten-year old student intending to strangle a classmate at school.
> Discussion about whether there is a more far-reaching threat scenario to consider.

The father of the family to which the ten-year old belongs has applied to the social services for protection of the family, as he suspects that one of his older sons plans to execute a man in a rival family to revenge a shooting that took place one year before this incident. If the murder is committed, the father expects retaliation. In retaliation for the earlier shooting, another of the father's sons has already been exposed to a revenge attack in which he was severely injured by gunfire and is now permanently wheelchair bound. This son has been placed in a protected residence because further threats against his life have been articulated by rival parties (the family is threatened by a dominant network in another PVA). The group discussed whether yet another criminal network from the other side of town might be involved in the conflict. According to the father, his son 'must' kill a member of the rival family network.

The meeting closed without any decisions about future actions being made. Instead, it had discussed how to label the issue: should it be called 'preparation for a criminal offence' or defined as a matter of 'conspiracy'? Since social services have an obligation to formally report any plans, they should also inform the father, but he was no longer contactable due to a change of phone number and an unknown address.

The requirement of working in a 'systematised' way in the sequence ordained by the CCP is not tailored to situations of this magnitude. Even the first step appeared difficult to manage at the observed meeting. How would one go about creating an overview of a situation as broad as this, in which different processes are intertwined in a way that pulling one string may have consequences far beyond what could be foreseen? Applying encoded knowledge (written rules and procedures) would obviously work up to a point, but what prevention strategy is to be injected into a chain where already precarious events have been retold and imbued with rumours and hearsay?

From our study, two strategies stand out. One would be to bureaucratize the case, letting routines and regulations, first and foremost from the police, guide further action. Such an approach would reduce uncertainty by making the situation manageable, but it does not provide any deeper understanding of the issues. This neutralising of uncertainty, and consequential frustration, may explain a general finding in our study about the police dependence in collaborative settings. This dependence can manifest as meetings being cancelled when not involving the police or being impeded or fettered in other ways. This implies that the adhocracy of the collaborative groups is sometimes dependant on the bureaucratic procedures of the dominant actor for the groups' functioning [27].

The other possible route, which especially some social workers spoke of as embodied knowledge, would be to have long experience of and personal relations with people living in the area. To call for this is to advocate for a kind of individual, domain-specific and autonomous knowledge (see Figure 1) [45] (p. 491). Since the meeting observed above had scarce knowledge resources of this kind at their disposal, they had to follow the first strategy or, as it turned out, they could not reach any collective strategy but halted at definitional issues. Generally, this strengthens previous research indicating a need for professionals embedded both in the public organisations and in the local community [25], and different forms of knowledge may be needed in conjunction.

6.3. Prevention as a Double-Edged Sword

Prevention following systematized steps in relation to possible threats of violence or acts of severe violence can also prove difficult because the steps may risk causing organizational or communication problems, or even result in yet more violence. The potential institutional logics—direction indicators coming out of the organization's design and knowledge types [46]—become fuzzy in collaboration. Moreover, the logics must be capable of preventing several potential 'ills' simultaneously and avoid future problems emanating from the solution itself.

When manifest violence has occurred, the groups are often faced with the delicate task of dealing with both the incident in itself and the question of how to communicate it to the public, as stated by the head of security in the area of A:

> Let's say for instance this weekend when we had a ... Well, we had a shooting this weekend and we found cartridges, cartridge cases. Communicating that part makes people scared of A. But the incident in itself is between two groups and has nothing to do with a third party. And it is very important that we communicate that this does not mean a risk for third parties, because it is between two groups, to sort of ... still create peace in the area. And it is delicate communication because this is not something we can ... We cannot communicate this on our website or the like, but it is word of mouth communication. (Head of security in A)

In this case, the issue of the shooting itself must be handled, as well as the possible consequence of people becoming scared of the residential area. The former issue could be dealt with through frank communication, but making people feel safe in the area may involve not communicating as frankly. What direction indicators [46] apply in such a dilemma? The orders of action are in conflict when it comes to managing communication: how can the group gain the necessary information to work with the incident while still keeping vital parts of the information private? In this case, the question of differences between individual and collective knowledge, or between tacit and explicit knowledge (see Figure 1), matters less, as it is seemingly an issue of working with an incidence of violence semi-covertly. However, once again, this makes the methodological order laid out by the CCP difficult to manage. The first step for surveying the problem becomes problematic if you must avoid making the inhabitants nervous while simultaneously carrying out an investigation.

Moreover, there are cases where the organizational logics appear not to be able to guide action because addressing a problem increases the risk of creating another problem. This is the case regardless of whether the actors are understood as separate entities belonging to each participating organization or are viewed as a group-specific conglomerate of diverging logics. In the extract below, the prevention group discussed a case where potential interventions to stop (sexual) violence would be likely to produce a risk of more violence.

> In one of the schools in the neighbourhood, a boy masturbated in front of a female teacher and molested her sexually by touching her body. The principal announced that she wanted to report the incident to the police. However, another teacher at the school shared information about the boy's family with the prevention group. According to this teacher, there was a high risk of a severe battery of the boy should the parents find out what had happened. As a result of this information, no report of concern about the boy was made to the social services.

To some extent, the situation above cannot be fitted into the matrix of professional actions recommended by the CCP. If they intervene, the professionals may ignite more violence; if they do nothing at all, the sexual violence is seemingly condoned. According to the logics within the police, the possibility of igniting violence would putatively not prevent a professional response, since the police's task is to uphold the law. For the social services, the teacher's warning about the possibility of a brutal assault by the parents of the boy would present a reason to set up a report of concern. In other words, the organizations involved in collaboration have already established institutional responses and explicit knowledge types (both encoded and embedded knowledge) ready for (at least parts of) this case. The patterns of actions are there, and thus should be of less concern for the CCP. Still, the meeting ends with no plans for action. In this situation, actions are supposed to take place through collaboration, but what is to be achieved or added *specifically* through collaboration is hard to see. Who would be the intended primary client or intervention object in the situation sketched: the molested teacher, the boy or the boy's parents? The answer appears to change depending on whether one asks the principal, the social services or the police.

Partnership approaches mean to assign an additional layer of (systematised) working orders that risk delaying the institutions' 'normal' responses that operate within each participating organization's collective knowledge [6]. Thus, instead of making work flows more effective, the result could be an obstruction of the operation of both collective and individual knowledge [45] (p. 491). The encoded knowledge type manifested in written rules and procedures [45] (p. 492–493), such as that delivered by the CCP, is in this event too simplified or too selective to be translated into concrete action. The same can be said about the embrained knowledge (based on theories and conceptual skills) behind the methods propagated by the CCP. In turn, this might in some instances mean that collaboration, as it is designed by the CCP, slows down the process of intervening.

7. Discussion

We've got a problem and we solve it through a collaborative meeting. And we meet, check, and it [the problem] is solved. But is it? (Security coordinator specialized at religious extremism in B)

The security coordinator quoted above points to the 'as if' problem of organizational action, i.e., the tendency to explain a certain action as if it has a particular effect, while this assumption is unfounded. Action is undertaken in line with what is thought of as adequate, and then dressed in the policy costume presently favoured [54]. In Sweden, there has been a strong inclination to call for collaborative action. However, there is a risk that this call is made without evidence that collaborative action has the capacity to handle issues better than individual organizational action, or that it can respond to the more difficult issues, such as aggravated violence or the challenges in PVAs. The organizational ideal of collaboration may turn out to be empty, with the risk of having it become a desirable end goal in itself.

Returning to the ontological dimension of knowledge as a matter of individual versus collective knowledge (see Figure 1) [45], we argue that there is a possibility that collaboration may become a knowledge form in itself. It may be understood as an individualistic form of knowledge, although surprisingly held by a group of individuals within the collaborative setting. Each group holds its 'own' knowledge, and in that sense, each group becomes a bounded rationality [50]. This knowledge, however, may not be centred around how to prevent severe violence but around how to execute collaboration. This particular skill becomes domain-specific and specialized, even if accumulated not within a single person but within a single constellation. Its relative success in combating school bullying, speeding on mopeds, battery or vandalism may simply be because the participating actors already possess organizational knowledge (or are familiar with the orders of action) on how these things are handled. However, lacking organizational methods to curb more brutish violence, such violence leaves the groups nonplussed.

In one sense, none of the knowledge models applied in analysis operate efficiently. This may at times be seen in the documents where details about the present situation in the area are to be merged into one document—the 'common operating scenarios' that the groups are to produce. These documents are to be generated once a week, and they form the basis for the efforts launched. They are perhaps the one artefact best summarising the difficulties that the groups face, as they are made to display information that ranges from 'mopeds speeding in the schoolyard' to 'murder committed outside the grocery store'. The knowledge that may explain two such very different events, and the knowledge underlying interventions addressing them, must inevitably differ. Embrained knowledge [45] (pp. 492–493) based on conceptual skills would obviously be useful, although difficult to balance in collaboration at the point where actors' different conceptual understandings must be merged. Embodied knowledge with its practical output may not be ideal, as it is carried by an individual. The encoded knowledge stored in rules and procedures might perhaps be the model best suited to the task. Still, one may ask: rules and procedures *for what?* In this case, are they more likely to revolve around rules for collaboration rather than procedures for intervention? The embedded knowledge based on an organization's joint understanding shares the same type of problem. Does this shared understanding orbit around ways to work together in the prescribed fashion, or is it applied to prevent crimes (murders) and promote security (making sure motor vehicles do not disturb the inhabitants)? The results in this study thus bear a relation to findings on other types of 'fuzzy' collaborative settings where group-decision is to take place. The strategies for inter-professional collaboration are often shaped by intuitive problem-solving [55], personal beliefs and experiences [56], dominating actors (leading to other actors submitting their beliefs) [57], a tendency to concentrate on orally conveyed details and initial impressions and to dismiss contradictory evidence [58], and a reliance on a collective memory of the group [59]. Adding a putative lack of a common goal as well as a lack of a joint knowledge base from which to operate, it is perhaps no wonder that one of the unarticulated organizational goals of the groups in question becomes precisely that: to collaborate.

Author Contributions: K.A. and T.F. both contributed equally to the design and implementation of the research, to the analysis of the results and to the writing of the manuscript. All authors have read and agreed to the published version of the manuscript.

Funding: Swedish Research Council for Health, Working Life and Welfare (FORTE). Registration no. 2018-01353.

Institutional Review Board Statement: The study was conducted according to the guidelines of the Declaration of Helsinki, and approved by the National Authority for Research Ethics (protocol code 2019-01858, 9 April 2019).

Informed Consent Statement: Informed consent was obtained from all subjects involved in the study. The study only involved professionals and did not cover any sensitive personal data.

Data Availability Statement: Data are not public according to ethical guidelines.

Conflicts of Interest: The authors declare no conflict of interest.

Notes

1. See: https://www.regeringen.se/rattsliga-dokument/departementsserien-och-promemorior/1996/01/ds-199659/.
2. See: https://regeringen.se/tillsammansmotbrott.
3. The project received funding from the research council FORTE. Ethical approval was requested, and an advisory statement obtained, Dnr: 2019-01858. Since the project does not involve sensitive personal data, it falls outside the legislation on research ethics.

References

1. McCave, E.L.; Rishel, C.W. Prevention as an explicit part of the social work profession: A systematic investigation. *Adv. Soc. Work* **2011**, *12*, 226–240. [CrossRef]
2. Sarnecki, J. *Stöta på Patrull—En ESO-Rapport om Polisens Problemorienterade Arbete. [Tackling Obstacles: An ESO Report on the Police's Problem-Oriented Work]*; Regeringskansliet: Stockholm, Sweden, 2019.
3. SOU. *Kommuner mot Brott. [Municipalities against CRIME]*; Elanders: Stockholm, Sweden, 2021; Volume 49.
4. Andersson, J. The Swedish National Council for Crime Prevention. A short presentation. *J. Scand. Stud. Criminol. Crime Prev.* **2005**, *6*, 74–88. [CrossRef]
5. Edvall Malm, D. *Det Socio-Polisiära Handlingsnätet: Om Kopplingar Mellan Polis och Socialtjänst Kring Ungdomars Kriminalitet och Missbruk. [The Socio-Police Action Net: On Connections between the Police and the Social Services in Cases of Youth Criminality and Drug Abuse]*; Umeå Universitet, Institutionen för Socialt Arbete: Stockholm, Sweden, 2012.
6. Forkby, T. Organisational Exceptions as Vehicles for Change: Collaborative strategies, trust, and counter strategies in local crime prevention partnerships in Sweden. *Eur. J. Soc. Work* **2020**, *23*, 580–593. [CrossRef]
7. Hallin, P.-O. *Effektiv Samordning av Brottsförebyggande och Trygghetsskapande Arbete i Socialt Utsatta Områden. [Effective Collaboration around Crime Prevention and Safety Promotion Efforts in Socially Disadvantaged Neighbourhoods]*; Urbana Studier, The University of Malmö: Malmö, Sweden, 2018; Available online: https://www.divaportal.org/smash/get/diva2:1410304/FULLTEXT01.pdf (accessed on 14 February 2022).
8. Johansson, K. Crime prevention cooperation in Sweden: A regional case study. *J. Scand. Stud. Criminol. Crime Prev.* **2014**, *14*, 143–158. [CrossRef]
9. Phillimore, J.; Humphries, R.; Klaas, F.; Knecht, M. Bricolage: Potential as a conceptual tool for understanding access to welfare in superdiverse neighbourhoods. In *IRIS Working Paper Series*; University of Birmingham: Birmingham, UK, 2016.

10. Sarnecki, J.; Carlsson, C. *Introduktion till Kriminologi. 2, Straff och Prevention. [Introduction to Criminology. 2. Punishment and Prevention]*; Studentlitteratur: Lund, Switzerland, 2021.

11. Takala, H. Nordic cooperation in criminal policy and crime prevention. *J. Scand. Stud. Criminol. Crime Prev.* **2004**, *5*, 131–147. [CrossRef]

12. Crawford, A. *Crime Prevention and Community Safety: Politics, Policies and Practices*; Longman: Harlow, UK, 1998.

13. Gilling, D. Community safety and social policy. *Eur. J. Crim. Policy Res.* **2001**, *9*, 381–400. [CrossRef]

14. Hughes, G.; Gilling, D. 'Mission impossible'? The habitus of the community safety manager and the new expertise in the local partnership governance of crime and safety. *Crim. Justice* **2004**, *4*, 129–149. [CrossRef]

15. Crawford, A.; Cunningham, M. Working in partnership: The challenges of working across organisational boundaries, cultures and practices. In *Police Leadership: Rising to the Top*; Fleming, J., Ed.; Oxford University Press: Oxford, UK, 2015; pp. 71–94.

16. Welsh, B.C.; Farrington, D.P. Evidence-based crime prevention. In *Preventing Crime. What Works for Children, Offenders, Victims and Places*; Springer: New York, NY, USA, 2007.

17. Braga, A.A. Policing crime hot spots. In *Preventing Crime. What Works for Children, Offenders, Victims and Places*; Welsh, B.C., Farrington, D.P., Eds.; Springer: New York, NY, USA, 2007.

18. Eck, J.E.; Clarke, R.V. Situational Crime Prevention: Theory, Practice and Evidence. In *Handbook on Crime and Deviance*; Marvin, D.K., Hendrix, N., Hall, G.P., Lizotte, A.J., Eds.; Springer: Cham, Swizerland, 2019.

19. Hope, T. Community crime prevention in Britain: A strategic overview. *Criminol. Crim. Justice* **2001**, *1*, 421–439. [CrossRef]

20. Fledderus, J.; Honingh, M. Why people co-produce within activation services: The necessity of motivation and trust—An investigation of selection biases in a municipal activation programme in the Netherlands. *Int. Rev. Adm. Sci.* **2016**, *82*, 69–87. [CrossRef]

21. Jakobsen, M. Can government initiatives increase citizen coproduction? Results of a randomized field experiment. *J. Public Adm. Res. Theory* **2013**, *23*, 27–54. [CrossRef]

22. Jakobsen, M.; Andersen, S.C. Coproduction and equity in public service delivery. *Public Adm. Rev.* **2013**, *73*, 704–713. [CrossRef]

23. Bannister, J.; Croudace, R.; Pickering, J.; Lightowler, C. Building safer communities: Knowledge mobilisation and community safety in Scotland. *Crime Prev. Community Saf.* **2011**, *13*, 232–245. [CrossRef]

24. Sutton, A.; Cherney, A. Prevention without politics? The cyclical progress of crime prevention in an Australian state. *Criminol. Crim. Justice* **2002**, *2*, 325–344. [CrossRef]

25. Bowden, M. Community safety, social cohesion and embedded autonomy: A case from south-west Dublin. *Crime Prev. Community Saf.* **2017**, *19*, 87–102. [CrossRef]

26. Harkin, D. Community safety partnerships: The limits and possibilities of 'policing with the community'. *Crime Prev. Community Saf.* **2018**, *20*, 125–136. [CrossRef]

27. Hope, T. The new local governance of community safety in England and Wales. *Can. J. Criminol. Crim. Justice* **2005**, *47*, 369–387. [CrossRef]

28. Bovaird, T.; Van Ryzin, G.G.; Loeffler, E.; Parrado, S. Activating citizens to participate in collective co-production of public services. *J. Soc. Policy* **2015**, *44*, 1–23. [CrossRef]

29. Bullock, K. Responding to anti-social behaviour: Analysis, interventions and the transfer of knowledge. *Crime Prev. Community Saf.* **2011**, *13*, 1–15. [CrossRef]

30. de Graaf, L.; van Hulst, M.; Michels, A. Enhancing participation in disadvantaged urban neighbourhoods. *Local Gov. Stud.* **2015**, *41*, 44–62. [CrossRef]

31. Braga, A.A.; Turchan, B.S.; Papachristos, A.V.; Hureau, D.M. Hot spots policing and crime reduction: An update of an ongoing systematic review and meta-analysis. *J. Exp. Criminol.* **2019**, *15*, 289–311. [CrossRef]

32. Piroozfar, P.; Farr, E.R.; Aboagye-Nimo, E.; Osei-Berchie, J. Crime prevention in urban spaces through environmental design: A critical UK perspective. *Cities* **2019**, *95*, 102411. [CrossRef]

33. Weisburd, D. Hot spots of crime and place-based prevention. *Criminol. Public Policy* **2018**, *17*, 5–25. [CrossRef]

34. Flemming, J.; Rhodes, R. Can experience be evidence? Craft knowledge and evidence-based policing. *Policy Polit.* **2018**, *46*, 3–26. [CrossRef]

35. Haggerty, K.D. From risk to precaution: The rationalities of personal crime prevention. In *Risk and Morality*; Doyle, A., Ericson, R.V., Eds.; Toronto University Press: Toronto, ON, Canada, 2003.

36. Armstead, T.L.; Wilkins, N.; Doreson, A. Indicators for evaluating community- and societal-level risk and protective factors for violence prevention: Findings from a review of the literature. *J. Public Health Manag. Pract.* **2019**, *24*, 42–50. [CrossRef]

37. Butts, J.A.; Roman, C.G.; Bostwick, L.; Porter, J.R. Cure violence: A public health model to reduce gun violence. *Annu. Rev. Public Health* **2015**, *36*, 39–53. [CrossRef]

38. Braga, A.A.; Weisburd, D.; Turchan, B. Focused deterrence strategies and crime control: An updated systematic review and meta-analysis of the empirical evidence. *Criminol. Public Policy* **2018**, *17*, 205–250. [CrossRef]

39. Ivert, A.; Mellgren, C.; Nilsson, J. *Processutvärdering av Sluta Skjut. [A Process Evaluation to Stop Shooting]*; Malmö Universitet: Malmö, Sweden, 2020.

40. Corsaro, N.; Engel, R.S. Community-based crime reduction in Tulsa: An application of Petersilia's multi-stakeholder collaborative approach to improve policy relevance and reduce crime risk. *Justice Q.* **2020**, *37*, 1199–1220. [CrossRef]

41. Petersilisa, J. Influencing public policy: An embedded criminologist reflects on California prison reform. *J. Exp. Criminol.* **2008**, *4*, 335–356. [CrossRef]
42. Matt, E. Commentary on community safety in Germany. *Crime Prev. Community Saf.* **2011**, *13*, 288–293. [CrossRef]
43. Recasens i Brunet, A.; Rodríguez Basanta, A. Development of the management of safety in Spain: Decentralisation with little organisation. *Crime Prev. Community Saf.* **2011**, *13*, 273–283. [CrossRef]
44. Clancey, G. A local case study of the crime decline. *Safer Communities* **2015**, *14*, 104–114. [CrossRef]
45. Lam, A. Tacit knowledge, organizational learning and social institutions: An integrated framework. *Organ. Stud.* **2000**, *21*, 487–515. [CrossRef]
46. Thornton, P.H.; Ocasio, W. Institutional logics. In *The Sage Handbook of Organizational Institutionalism*; Greenwood, R., Ed.; SAGE: London, UK, 2008.
47. Hodgson, D. Project work: The legacy of bureaucratic control in the post-bureaucratic organization. *Organization* **2004**, *11*, 81–100. [CrossRef]
48. Birkinshaw, J.; Ridderstråle, J. Adhocracy for an agile age. *McKinsey Q.* **2015**, *4*, 44–57. Available online: http://search.ebscohost.com.proxy.lnu.se/login.aspx?direct=true&db=bsu&AN=112963953&site=ehost-live (accessed on 27 January 2022).
49. Mintzberg, H.; McHugh, A. Strategy formation in an adhocracy. *Adm. Sci. Q.* **1985**, *30*, 160–197. [CrossRef]
50. Simon, H. *Administrative Behaviour*; Macmillan: New York, NY, USA, 1957.
51. Walsh, J.P.; Ungson, G.R. Organizational Memory. *Acad. Manag. Rev.* **1991**, *16*, 57–91. [CrossRef]
52. Brown, J.S.; Duguid, P. Organizational learning and communities of practice: Towards a unified view of working, learning and innovation. *Organ. Sci.* **1991**, *2*, 40–57. [CrossRef]
53. BRÅ. *Det Brottsförebyggande Arbetet i Sverige. Nuläge och Utvecklingsbehov. [Crime Prevention in Sweden: Present Situation and Development Needs]*; Brottsförebyggande Rådet: Stockholm, Sweden, 2021.
54. DiMaggio, P.; Powell, W. The iron cage revisited: Institutional isomorphism and collective rationality in organizational fields. *Am. Sociol. Rev.* **1983**, *48*, 147–160. [CrossRef]
55. van de Luitgaarden, G.M.J. Evidence-based practice in social work: Lessons from judgement and decision-making theory. *Br. J. Soc. Work* **2009**, *39*, 243–260. [CrossRef]
56. Dellgran, P.; Höjer, S. *Forskning i Praktiken. Om den Seniora Forskningens Innehåll och Socionomers Forskningsorientering [Research in Practice. The Content of Senior Research and Social Workers' Research Orientation]*; National Agency for Higher Education: Stockholm, Sweden, 2003.
57. Prince, J.; Gear, A.; Jones, C.; Read, M. The child protection conference: A study of process and an evaluation of the potential for on-line group support. *Child Abus. Rev.* **2005**, *14*, 113–131. [CrossRef]
58. Munroe, E. Common errors of reasoning in child protection work. *Child Abus. Negl.* **1999**, *23*, 745–758. [CrossRef]
59. Forkby, T.; Höjer, S. Navigations between regulations and gut instinct: The unveiling of collective memory in decision-making processes where teenagers are placed in residential care. *Child Fam. Soc. Work* **2011**, *16*, 159–168. [CrossRef]

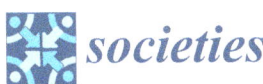

societies

MDPI

Article

The Feasibility and Acceptability of an Experience-Based Co-Design Approach to Reducing Domestic Abuse

Shoshana Gander-Zaucker [1,*], Gemma L. Unwin [1] and Michael Larkin [2]

1   School of Psychology, University of Birmingham, Birmingham B15 2TT, UK; g.l.unwin@bham.ac.uk
2   Institute of Health and Neurodevelopment, Aston University, Birmingham B4 7ET, UK; m.larkin@aston.ac.uk
*   Correspondence: sxg589@alumni.bham.ac.uk

Abstract: One means of reducing violence against people experiencing domestic abuse is to improve the pathway which they use to access help from the police and other services. In this paper we report and reflect on a project which contributes to violence reduction via a participatory approach to service improvement, focusing on this pathway. We describe the four phases of an innovative experience-based co-design (EBCD) project, which involved collaborating with domestic abuse survivors as well as members of the police and domestic abuse organizations. We report on indicators of the acceptability and feasibility of EBCD in this context. We also reflect upon the potential of the EBCD approach for involving communities in collaborating with services to reduce domestic abuse. We discuss the conceptual and methodological implications with regard to adopting participatory and inclusive approaches in contexts where power-sharing may be difficult. We argue that EBCD has considerable potential for use in this setting and we identify several areas where insights from this project could be used to improve the future viability of any such initiatives.

Keywords: violence; domestic abuse; co-design; acceptability; feasibility; epistemic justice; help-seeking; service improvement; police; independent domestic violence advisors

Citation: Gander-Zaucker, S.; Unwin, G.L.; Larkin, M. The Feasibility and Acceptability of an Experience-Based Co-Design Approach to Reducing Domestic Abuse. *Societies* **2022**, *12*, 93. https://doi.org/10.3390/soc12030093

Academic Editors: Jaimee Mallion and Erika Gebo

Received: 19 March 2022
Accepted: 9 June 2022
Published: 15 June 2022

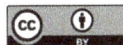
1. Introduction

The World Health Organization estimates that 1 in 3 women globally are affected by domestic abuse in their lifetimes [1]. Domestic abuse-related crimes include the occurrence of threatening behavior, violence, or abuse (physical, psychological, emotional, sexual, financial) between intimate partners or family members, who are aged 16 years and over, regardless of gender or sexuality [2]. The Crime Survey for England and Wales ending March 2020 evaluated that 5.5% of adults aged 16 to 74 years (2.3 million) experienced domestic abuse in the previous 12 months [3], which is an estimated 7.3% of women and 3.6% of men [4]. In the year ending March 2021, 18% of all offences recorded by the police in England and Wales were domestic abuse-related crimes and prevalence is increasing, rising 6% from the prior year. [3] Domestic violence is not typically an isolated event: case study analyses consistently show recurrent patterns of abusive behavior (e.g., see Katerndahl et al. [5]).

One way to reduce violence against people experiencing domestic abuse is to improve the acceptability and effectiveness of the help-seeking pathway. Prevailing models of help-seeking tend to characterize the problem as an issue of individual knowledge, self-appraisal, and reasoned action [6]. Domestic abuse is an important context here because the problem and pathway are complex. The problem is complex because identifying and accepting that abuse is taking place, in the context of a familial or intimate relationship, can be difficult. Deciding to seek help may be shaped by a range of cultural, social, and relational factors [7], and by the opportunity, knowledge, and access required in order to approach someone who can help [8]. The pathway is also complex because it is provided by a range of organizations, with different interests (e.g., support and safety; housing and security; law and order; risk and child welfare), whose collaborative arrangements are varied, and opaque to the help-seeker. Some of these organizations have limited or unstable funding, and some may have different 'thresholds' for providing help. The help which a person hopes for may not be the help that they are most likely to receive

A report by a UK-based domestic abuse charity highlighted that many survivors went to the police multiple times before obtaining effective help [9]. It is crucial that domestic abuse survivors receive help which they find effective when they first seek it, because at the point when a survivor obtains help, the abuse may be escalating in either severity, frequency, or both [9]. This can have serious and negative implications for their safety [9]. Furthermore, survivors who are satisfied with police services and find their services helpful are more likely to contact the police again, if needed [10]. Therefore, it is important to understand what survivors find helpful and unhelpful when seeking help and to design services to meet these needs. One way of achieving this is by involving domestic abuse survivors in service development. This would ensure that services are tailored to domestic abuse survivors' views and real needs and therefore improve the help-seeking pathway both for survivors and service providers.

This paper reports and reflects on an attempt to contribute to violence reduction via a collaborative community-based approach to service improvement, called experience-based co-design (EBCD [11]). EBCD is a participatory, action research process, which was originally developed as a tool for improving patient and staff experiences of healthcare services [12]. Co-design is a form of community-based action which involves working closely with stakeholder groups to make shared decisions about how to improve a common resource, important process, or shared environment. EBCD is a relatively formalized approach to co-design, with accessible steps and strategies, which can be implemented in public services. As a result, it is becoming an increasingly important tool in the development of such services [13,14]. Here we aim to contribute to the field of violence reduction by reporting on a novel implementation of EBCD in this context, and to the development of EBCD itself, by discussing the approach in the context of a conceptual framework which helps us to consider how EBCD work shifts the traditional relationship between 'service provider' and 'service user'.

EBCD has been used in a range of community contexts (physical healthcare, mental healthcare, learning disability, interventions research) to collaboratively create a wide range of 'things'—information resources, service improvements, built environments, implementation pathways (e.g., see Dimopoulos-Bick et al.'s synthesis [15], and Donetto et al.'s review [13]). For example, a survey has found that EBCD projects have been undertaken in the following range of clinical services: cancer, diabetes, genetics, drug and alcohol services, intensive care, emergency services, palliative care, orthopedics, surgical units, hematology, and neonatal and pediatric care [13]. The findings of the survey have also demonstrated that at the time it was conducted, EBCD projects were either achieved or being conducted in the following countries: UK, Canada, New Zealand, Australia, Sweden, and the Netherlands [13].

EBCD has not previously been implemented in the context of policing and domestic abuse and so our primary purpose in this paper is to describe the process that we undertook, and to reflect upon the acceptability and feasibility [16] of this approach for community-based approaches which involve a range of partner-organizations. Thus, the project described here increases our knowledge of how EBCD works, for whom, and in what contexts, especially surrounding the issues involving domestic abuse. This paper aims to answers the research question, 'Is it feasible and acceptable to conduct EBCD in the field of domestic violence?'.

Our project took place in a major conurbation in England. The conurbation is ethnically diverse. It has been undergoing a long transition from an economy based on heavy industry to a much more mixed economy. It was jointly commissioned by a Police and Crime Commissioners Office and a local police force. The project was initially commissioned to explore satisfaction of domestic abuse survivors with their services and to use these findings to provide recommendations for service improvements. The local police force approached researchers at the University of Birmingham in 2015 with proposals for a survey of domestic abuse survivors. Through discussion with representatives of the police force, it was agreed instead to use an EBCD framework, first to understand the experiences of survivors, and then to collaboratively plan service developments. As partial funding came from the local police force, the study was based in the region covered by its service.

EBCD begins with a phase of finding out about people's experience of a particular process or environment. These insights are organized as 'touchpoints'—features of an environment or process that make a difference to people's experience. EBCD then moves to a 'feedback' phase, which involves consulting with the different stakeholder groups to discuss the touchpoints and generate consensus about what needs to change. These stakeholder groups may include patients, staff, and carers. It concludes with a co-design phase, where the different stakeholders work together to decide how to make improvements, and who should make them. In this way, the different stakeholders in a given community work together to identify things which could be improved, and they continue to collaborate in order to decide how to make those improvements.

An EBCD approach prompts us to reflect upon help-seeking as a systemic and relational activity precisely because it brings together different stakeholders. The involvement of survivors from different communities prompts us to consider accessibility and knowledge. The involvement of different elements of police services (e.g., specialist and generic; call handling and first response) prompts us to return to the question of knowledge from a service perspective, and to consider it in the context of communication with help-seekers, and the consistency and empathy of the response. The involvement of third-sector services brings the issue of communication *between* services into view. When we consider these different groups as members of a community of people who are collectively 'responding to domestic abuse', we see a shared value: *domestic abuse is wrong, and something should be done about it*. However, we also see a range of different views about which actions to prioritize in responding to that.

It is certainly possible to imagine a community-based EBCD project which does not involve the police as key partners, but in this project, the police played an important role. In many ways, this was positive—the nature of policing organizations is such that they have high standards for governance, internal organization, and project management. These assisted with recruitment and engagement to the project, and with subsequent commitments to implementing the project's recommendations. However, it is also important to consider the implications of police involvement upon a method which is committed to collaboration and community-led change.

Epistemic justice [17] is a conceptual framework which is helpful in this regard, and which can help us to think more generally about the dynamics of coproduction—and particularly some of the complexities involved in implementing a community-based approach when some community-members (i.e., perpetrators) are deliberately excluded from the work [18,19] and where other community-members (i.e., police) hold considerably more power than the vulnerable population at the center of the work [13]. This conceptual framework approaches the question of knowledge from a philosophical perspective which is concerned with equality and justice. For example, knowledge about what to call a problem, how to identify it, and what to do when you encounter it. There are some direct and immediately helpful entailments, in terms of the way that Fricker's terminology conceptualizes the disadvantages and injustices experienced by those survivors of violence who are—for example—situated in social and cultural environments which do not consider intimate partner violence to be unacceptable, or which grant spousal perpetrators certain exceptions, or which understand help-seeking from outsiders to be shameful. These are all forms of hermeneutic injustice, because they involve a person who is disadvantaged by knowledge that they do not have or cannot access. Similarly, Fricker's concept of testimonial injustice applies to the many situations in which survivors of violence are not believed due to the biases of the person from whom they seek help: they may not be believed by in-laws, for example, because the perpetrators are family members; or by the police, because the survivors are either from communities where domestic abuse is not expected, or conversely, is not problematized by the police. Therefore, our secondary purpose in this paper is to reflect on some of the workings of a co-design approach to domestic abuse through the lens of epistemic justice, and a means of considering its potential contribution to harm reduction. This framework was not used to *plan* our implementation of the study. We followed the standard pragmatic process of EBCD. However, we have found it useful as a means of reflecting on what happens *during* the implementation of EBCD work, and of linking to established models of the acceptability of interventions [20]. This paper therefore outlines the methods used in each stage of the project with accompanying reflections on the acceptability and feasibility of those methods, followed by a discussion on the overall process and potential impact of the study, drawing on the existing literature.

2. Our Project

The project started early in 2016 and was guided by a steering group, gathered together by the local police force, with guidance from the research group, and including representation from police. It was usually comprised of two police officers, one of them the senior officer acting as project lead from within the police; two domestic abuse survivors; the lead for local authority's co-ordinating domestic abuse organization, and the research team (n = 2–3). The group met once every two to three months for the lifespan of the project and meetings were usually chaired by the senior police officer.

The group set and followed an agenda, but the chair took care to actively invite contributions from all the different stakeholders. As a result, many of the challenges this project faced were resolved through this group. Thus, when the research team felt 'stuck' with something, the other members of the steering group would furnish them with a new set of strategies. For example, this occurred when trying to recruit participants for the project. Furthermore, the insights of the survivors, police officers, and support lead on the steering group were invaluable. For example, their help was especially important when it came to designing the interview schedules, developing recruitment strategies, reviewing the touchpoints from the research phase, and assisting in planning and running the co-design event. Consequently, this had a positive impact on the outcome of the research project. For example, they greatly helped in recruiting participants and ensured that the interview schedules were sensitive to participants' needs.

The EBCD project was conducted in four phases, described in detail in the following sections. See Figure 1 for an overview of the process. The first two phases focused on stakeholders within one city in central England. These stakeholders included domestic abuse survivors, representatives of the police, and independent domestic violence advisors (IDVAs) who provide specialist support to survivors. To increase participation, the latter two phases expanded the range to include stakeholders from the wider region but still within acceptable travel times to allow in-person meetings. The first phase, which acted as the research phase, involved gathering experiences of providing or using services to generate a list of 'touchpoints' or features of this process which had an impact on how it was experienced. In this project, we decided to refer to touchpoints as keypoints, because survivors preferred it. In the second phase, in which the feedback groups were conducted, we brought together groups of stakeholders to further discuss the touchpoints and to prioritize areas for action. The third phase involved the co-design event where stakeholders came together and engaged in solution-focused discussion to generate action plans. In the final stage of the project, which acted as the implementation phase, the police were responsible for observing and implementing these action plans. The figure below describes the phases of the project, their aims, and who was involved. It is here to set the scene for the detailed description which will follow and thus enhances our understanding of how the project advanced from one stage to the other.

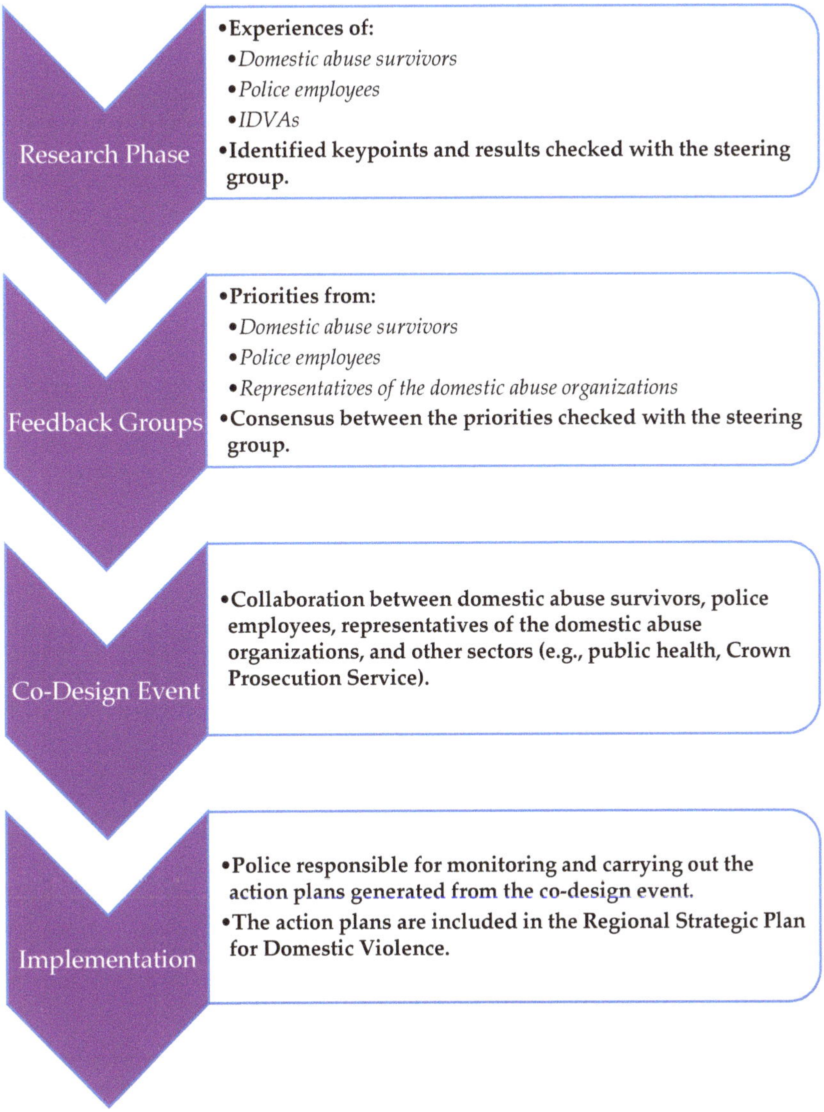

Figure 1. Overview of the EBCD project.

2.1. The Research Phase

- *Recruitment*

The aim of the research phase was to gather the experiences of domestic abuse survivors, the police, and the IDVAs. We set out to recruit service providers (which included representation from the police and IDVAs) and domestic abuse survivors, who could provide personal experiential perspectives on the pathway for accessing and receiving help. Domestic abuse survivors were eligible to participate if they had experienced domestic abuse within the past 24 months. We aimed to include a diverse range of perspectives. We used purposive sampling to pursue this. In the case of service providers, purposive sampling allowed us to ensure that we included participants with a wide range of roles. In the case of service users, we included participants with a range of ethnic backgrounds, and with a range of differing relationships to the perpetrator.

Domestic abuse survivors were recruited via gatekeepers from domestic abuse support organizations and the police force in the city. Service providers were eligible to participate if they were involved as a professional in a service provided by a support organization or the police force of the county this project was conducted for. The service providers were recruited with the assistance of the members of the steering group, who were involved in the services provided by either the police or the domestic abuse organizations.

- *Data collection*

We conducted either semi-structured face-to-face individual interviews or focus group discussions, in English, with our participants. Most of them were carried out by the authors, but a small number were carried out with support from master's students. Both the interviews and the focus groups were open-ended data collection events, facilitated by an interviewer drawing on a set of exploratory questions in a topic guide. The questions in the topic guide were generated by consulting with representatives of all stakeholders at the steering group. Thus, we prepared schedules of open-ended questions to explore participants' experiences of the help-seeking process, and we employed these flexibly, following established standards for semi-structured approaches to qualitative data collection [21].

Data collection lasted 14 months; the service users were interviewed during an eight-month period within that window. We continued to try to recruit service users for the remaining period of four months but were unable to increase our sample size. It proved to be challenging to recruit survivors for the project due to the vulnerability of the survivors and potentially changes in the circumstances of survivors who showed initial interest in participating.

The interviews lasted 41–121 min. Focus groups lasted approximately two hours. All of the interviews and focus groups were audio-recorded in full and transcribed verbatim.

- *Participants*

Six survivors (five women; one man), participated in this phase of the project. All the survivors were parents, had received services from an organization which supports domestic abuse survivors, and had suffered from multiple incidents of abuse. The abuse had occurred within a context of a heterosexual relationship.

Twenty-two police participants took part across ten individual interviews and three focus groups, including seven senior police officers. They included: initial response police officers, non-urgent and urgent call handlers, force contact management, dispatch and resource allocation staff, offender management, specialist police officers working for the Public Protection Unit who investigate domestic abuse offences, and those involved in policy and strategy related to domestic abuse.

Three IDVAs, all women, participated across one individual interview and one group discussion. One IDVA was a court IDVA. A fourth, male participant, was a service delivery officer. For the purposes of brevity, we will refer to them as IDVAs.

Interpretation of data in EBCD is often conducted relatively informally [11] but there are also some advantages to taking a more formalized and systematic approach [22]. In this project, the authors analyzed full transcripts of the interviews. We identified keypoints using an inductive, open coding strategy in the manner of the early stages of a thematic analysis. From the transcripts, we systematically extracted each claim that was made about the valence of an experience (e.g., whether it was good or bad), alongside a code about what this meant to the participant, and then recorded all of this information in a coding framework. Rather than developing 'themes' per se, after reviewing all of the extracted keypoints, we sorted them into groups based on their shared concerns and translated each group into a single paraphrased statement. The identified keypoints are listed in Table 1, below.

Table 1. List of the keypoints drawn from the accounts of the participants [1].

Keypoints Drawn from the Accounts of the Survivors, Police Employees, and IDVAs
• Services need to be ready to support people who will have different 'tipping points' for seeking help.
• Services need to be ready to support people who have had 'help' imposed upon them.
• Services need to be ready to support people who want different sorts of solutions.
• The police are perceived to be ineffective, or even make things worse.
• The police will not understand.
• It can be difficult to get/find help.
• All professionals need to be aware that children, or the relationship with the children, may be put at risk.
• Organizations can leave survivors feeling excluded from their processes.
• Positive contact can help survivors to feel safe and reassured.
• Once other people were involved, their support/involvement was often very helpful to survivors.
• It is perceived to be difficult to get effective help when your problem does not fit the mold.
• It is vital for the police to get good information in order to tailor their response.
• A good response is a prompt and effective response.
• Police work is psychologically taxing—relatively informal resources are used to support this.
• Some practices can undermine people's willingness to return to the police for help.
• Organizations can be poor at communicating with each other.
• There are tools which are not always used or are not available everywhere or are not effective.
• It can be difficult for the police to know how to make a difference in domestic abuse cases.
• It is important to educate the public about abusive behavior.

[1] *We do not provide a detailed presentation of the findings from the research phase of this project in this paper, because our aim here is to give an overview of the approach that we took, and to share our insights with regard to its acceptability and feasibility for harm reduction approaches directly involving communities.*

The findings from the research phase highlighted that domestic abuse survivors could find it difficult to get/find support that was sensitive to their needs from the police and domestic abuse organizations. Their negative experiences of help-seeking were seen as undermining their willingness to return to the police for help. The police recognized that their services were variable and that unfortunately not all survivors received a good response and therefore that poor services *do* need to improve. The police and IDVA participants acknowledged that survivors might want cases to be resolved in different ways (e.g., some survivors might want the perpetrator locked up, while others might want to stay in the relationship but to have the abuse stop). Another important area of focus of discussion for all three stakeholder groups was around the importance of communication. For example, the domestic abuse survivors highlighted that it was important to them that there was good communication between them and their formal service providers. Similarly, service providers spoke about the importance of good communication in their work. The IDVAs were frustrated that although they shared information with the police, the police did not always do the same with them.

In EBCD, the identification of touchpoints/keypoints is an important step in providing focus to the co-design work. The keypoints act as a stimulus for further conversations about what should change, and how it should change, during the remaining phases. Crucially, this still leaves space for the inclusion of new perspectives (in our case, both additional survivors, and wider professional perspectives), and further refinement of the co-design community's aims.

Interim Discussion: Indicators of Acceptability and Feasibility during Recruitment and Engagement

It is important to reflect on the acceptability and feasibility of this phase of the project for potential further initiatives. It was certainly feasible to recruit service providers to this project: both police and IDVAs were quick to understand the project, and soon engaged with the research phase. There was often a good initial response from survivors too. Many expressed an interest in taking part, but when it came to arranging interviews, there were often difficulties in making contact with survivors, in setting up suitable interview arrangements, or in survivors attending the interview. We were not able to collect substantive feedback on why these difficulties arose, but through discussion with various stakeholders on the steering group and beyond, we tried a range of alternative strategies to invite and involve survivors as research participants. A further challenge stemmed from some survivors being in too vulnerable a situation to participate (e.g., due to concerns that the perpetrator would find out). Allowing for eligibility of service users to participate for a longer period after the abuse had occurred would have helped with this. Services themselves had little time to support recruitment of participants, but there was better engagement when they were able to do this. From the perspective of the epistemic justice framework, these issues underline the power differentials which are in play during the opening round of a co-design project. Projects may reproduce or amplify hermeneutic injustices, because service users do not *know* what the process will involve, or what will be asked of them, prompting wariness about getting involved. If their prior experience of the services has been poor, it may fuel *expectations* of testimonial injustice—that they will not be believed. Trust is clearly crucial in this context.

The data collected also had several limitations. First, four of the domestic abuse survivors agreed to be interviewed in English but were not as fluent in English as they were in their first languages. The project did not include funding for interpreters, but these participants may have been able to express themselves more comfortably, and more eloquently, if we had been able to use interpreters. Second, all the survivors participating in the first phase of the project had sought help, lived in the same region of the UK, and had children. The sample only included one male participant. We tried to compensate for this by including the perspectives of service providers who described the needs of other male survivors. This does mean that our starting sample did not account for the full diversity of survivors of domestic abuse. However, the data collected had two key strengths. First, they successfully captured the participants' lived experiences of help-seeking/providing support, as well as the impact these experiences had on them. Second, for a qualitative study, where the focus typically prioritizes depth over breadth [21], it included a relatively large sample of service providers.

2.2. The Feedback Group Phase

In EBCD, the primary purpose of these groups is to discuss, cluster, and prioritize the keypoints, in order that key areas of consensus can be taken forward to the co-design stage. An important secondary function is that these groups support perspective-taking: they allow stakeholders to see what other groups have said, and to prepare for the collaborative work of the co-design event. The groups also widen the range of perspectives involved in the process, expanding out beyond the initial interview sample. We conducted 12 feedback groups with approximately 40 participants. At the end of each feedback event, the outcome was a list of the clustered and prioritized keypoints, as these were arranged by the stakeholders. We recorded these priorities in a spreadsheet and mapped the areas of agreement across the feedback events.

2.2.1. Results of the Feedback Groups

This produced five priority areas of consensus: (1) Having an open mind about who needs help and being ready to provide a humane first contact; (2) A range of options for responding which do not place further burdens on the survivor or their children; (3) Developing support and training for police officers; (4) Improving knowledge about when and where to seek help, and what to expect; (5) Improving information sharing and collaboration across organizations. The first four areas of consensus were identified by all stakeholder groups. In other words, they were identified by the survivors, police, and support organizations. The fifth area was primarily prioritized by the police and the support organizations but was also evidenced by the survivors.

2.2.2. Interim Discussion: Indicators of Acceptability and Feasibility during Feedback Events

During this stage it was comparatively easy to recruit participants from all stakeholder groups. We began to widen our geographical range, from city to region, for some of the feedback events. However, for survivors it may well also have helped that in this phase they could attend events *together*. This underlines the relational context of epistemic justice: it is therefore important in planning co-design to consider the dynamics involved in co-design activities. Setting up events with a collective service user presence may reduce the perceived threat of testimonial injustices. This observation is reflected in the wider coproduction literature. In addition, participants did not have to talk about their personal experiences to take part in these events, further reducing the potential inequities or anticipated challenges which might have discouraged participation in the previous phase.

Participating in this stage of the project appeared to be generally easier and more acceptable for survivors. On reflection, a *collective* means of participating in the research phase, rather than individual interviews, may have been helpful for engagement. However, our priority in adopting interviews for the first phase was to use a medium which would allow us to provide sensitive responses to any disclosures of risk or distress.

2.3. The Co-Design Event

The third phase of the co-design project was the co-design event. The co-design event took place at another university in the host city. An academic setting was chosen partly because it represented 'neutral ground,' and partly because the police wanted to highlight the strong academic emphasis that had been put into the project and the fact that it was conducting innovative work. The research team took the lead in organizing the co-design event but consulted with the other members of the steering group to do so effectively. For example, the members of the steering group decided together on the venue, as well as on whom to invite, but the research team hired the venue and sent out the invitations. In this project, the co-design event was very important since it brought all the stakeholders together to design an action plan to improve services based on the consensus areas. Forty people attended the co-design event. It developed around five working groups, with each of them focusing on one of the different consensus areas. Each group was assigned a facilitator, to keep the group 'on task', and a 'champion' to provide organizational advice on how plans could be implemented, and by whom. The facilitators were chosen by the steering group as those they personally knew from work and considered to have the best skills to fulfil this role. Furthermore, the champions were chosen by the steering group because they were people with organizational roles which would enable them to bring the action plans forward due to their senior positions and responsibilities. The aim of the co-design event was to create a space in which domestic abuse survivors and service providers could work collaboratively to design action plans to improve services. Therefore, mixed groups were created around each of the consensus areas. To support the action planning, groups were provided with a simple template, prompting them to record their aim, the steps needed to execute their plan, and an evaluation plan (how they would know when they had achieved it). Following this work, the groups were invited to share their plans in a series of short presentations.

2.3.1. Results of the Co-Design Event

Each of the five working groups produced at least one action plan. Some groups produced more than one plan, and some groups coordinated their plans to complement the work of other groups. A total of seven plans were proposed. These are briefly reviewed below in Table 2, according to working group.

Table 2. Proposed action plans according to working group.

Working Group	Proposed Action Plan
Group 1: *Having an open mind about who needs help and being ready to provide a humane first contact*	Proposal to improve survivor experience by providing more specialist support, with trial of domestic abuse specialist car (as per mental health triage team; police officer to be accompanied by peer support worker or IDVA) to provide timely follow-up to the first response.
Group 2: *A range of options for responding which do not place further burdens on the survivor or their children*	This group proposed two action plans: • To reduce risk to survivor by sharpening focus on perpetrators through more routine discussions and monitoring of perpetrators at multi-agency meetings. • To give safe period of reflection, post-first response, to the survivor, by development and trial of 'brief stay' respite accommodation for perpetrators, staffed with specialist worker.
Group 3: *Developing support and training for police officers*	Proposal to reduce variability of first responses by providing mandatory training to all response officers; this training would be delivered by a range of media (including face-to-face and survivor-led) to improve their understanding of the complexities underpinning domestic abuse, and the range of appropriate responses available to them.
Group 4: *Improving knowledge about when and where to seek help, and what to expect*	This group proposed two action plans: • To improve help-seeking in the longer-term by improving young people's knowledge about healthy relationships with a campaign/education program in schools. • For a survivor-informed review of currently available information (about domestic abuse and the help which is on offer) to identify areas for improvement.
Group 5: *Improving information sharing and collaboration across organizations*	Proposal to improve access to support by mapping the available services and tools, and then developing an online resource that provides details of different pathways and the help available at different points on those pathways, produced to link directly to relevant agency websites.

The underlying priority areas provide useful context for thinking about how these plans might be implemented, extended, given a sharper focus, or supplemented by further initiatives. For example, the group briefed to develop support and training for police officers focused on trying to improve consistency of first responses by proposing mandatory training on domestic abuse. However, they also had support in their remit, and there was considerable discussion during the feedback groups about the pressures of staff wellbeing, and the lack of available support after exposure to trauma or stress. Although this group found staff well-being an important topic, they did not design any action plans for this, but only created action plans for the training component. In retrospect, it might have been better to separate this group into two with one group focusing on staff training and the other on staff well-being.

2.3.2. Interim Discussion: Indicators of Acceptability and Feasibility during Co-Design Event

During the event we observed collaboration and communication between the different stakeholders, both within and between the working groups. The impact of survivor testimony was powerful, and clearly influenced the discussion and direction of each group's work.

At the end of the co-design event, feedback from the participants was gathered through an open-ended evaluation form. Although the form was anonymous, the participants could indicate if the feedback came from a survivor, family member, police employee, support professional, or another role. They could tick more than one option (e.g., if they were a survivor who also had a professional role in a support organization). Twenty-three of the forty participants completed the feedback form. Overall, the feedback from the event was excellent. The participants indicated that the presentations, which were held during the event, were interesting, easy to follow, and respectful of everyone's point-of-view. Furthermore, the groupwork also received positive comments with participants indicating that: it was easy to understand what they had to do; the group leaders kept everyone involved and on track; it was respectful of everyone's point-of-view; and useful since they came up with a plan that could make a difference. Moreover, the responses of the service providers indicated that: obtaining the feedback of domestic abuse survivors gave them a better insight; it helped pinpoint areas for improvement; they would like to take what they learned into their work; it was productive to have different perspectives at the table; the working groups were balanced in terms of stakeholders; and they hoped that the ideas that they generated would become a reality. On a less positive note, the feedback from some of the service providers also indicated that although the co-design event generated good ideas it was difficult to formulate the steps needed to execute them and there was not enough time to do so during the event either (the groups had an hour and 40 min to do so, which included a ten-minute break). The feedback from the survivors specified that they appreciated hearing the views of police employees, especially those of call handlers and initial response officers, and that they hoped that it would make a difference in the field of domestic abuse. By this stage, the co-design process appeared to be highly acceptable to stakeholders from all groups.

The steering group met once following the co-design event to discuss their observations from the event, the feedback that was obtained, and the handover of the final report. Following this meeting, the research team wrote a short report about the EBCD project for the police. The interim report summarized the process and recommendations from the co-design component. For example, it included the procedure of the whole project, the identified keypoints, results of the co-design event, and illustrative anonymized quotes of the participants. The report also included the feedback of the domestic abuse survivors who were part of the steering group about the process of being involved in an EBCD project. They provided a personal statement, which is included in Table 3, below.

Table 3. What is it like to be a survivor involved with an EBCD project?

What Is It Like to Be a Survivor Involved with an EBCD Project?
"As a survivor I have found being part of this research a huge success. I have been able to share my story of domestic abuse and how it has affected myself and my children, highlighting things that went well and things that went wrong. I have been able to rebuild positive relationships with many people working in the very service I had felt let down by. This process has been hard at times—opening up about difficult experiences. However, I believe this has contributed massively to my healing journey in a positive way. I have become much more confident at public speaking and this is helping me a great deal in my [title] degree".
"Being part of this research project has played a major role in my healing and recovery. Just knowing that it will benefit other survivors/victims, throughout different organizations, made it worthwhile and something that I not only wanted to do but felt I needed to do. I experienced some truly shocking responses from different organizations that were meant to help, so the chance to try and correct that for others wasn't one to be missed. I am really proud of the work and the dedication from the team. I hope that with it we can make a difference and others will receive the correct help that I so desperately needed".

These powerful comments from survivors who were involved with the project [23] show how a sense of shared enterprise may arise from being involved in a community-based participatory approach. Here, there is also a sense that participation in the co-design process may also contribute to people's own recovery journeys. These comments underscore the moral value of helping to make a difference, and how that comes with some personal cost, but they also show why it is so important that organizations *act* upon the outcomes of such processes.

2.4. Implementation

In this project, funding and research governance did not extend to the implementation stage. The police took responsibility for monitoring and carrying out the action plans generated from the co-design event. The action plans were subsequently included in the Regional Strategic Plan for Domestic Violence. We do not have data on which plans *were* then implemented, or how they were perceived to improve help-seeking experiences and contribute to harm reduction. We consider that it has been useful and important to show that this kind of approach *can* be conducted with the police as partners, and that it is acceptable and feasible for stakeholders in the field of domestic abuse. Further work is required to enhance the sustainability of EBCD approaches, and to provide evidence of subsequent improvements to services, in this context. This work should include structured study of the implementation processes following on from co-design.

3. Discussion

3.1. Implications

Previous authors have observed that providing more training does not in itself lead to direct improvements in policing [14]. To improve responses to meet the needs of survivors, culture change and behavior change are required. This project has shown that it is acceptable and feasible to involve those with a lived experience (of domestic abuse) in community-based collaborative approaches to improving services and reducing harm. Threats to feasibility were overcome. However, the project faced some problems of acceptability and feasibility, especially when it came to recruiting domestic abuse survivors for the research phase. In the preceding sections, we have discussed some ways in which this issue could be resolved to promote greater community involvement at all phases of the project.

Taken together, our observations from the final co-design stage suggest that this critical step in the EBCD approach to community involvement was highly acceptable to participants. It seems that by this final stage of the EBCD process, further improvements had been made with regard to the epistemic inequalities and injustices which initially hampered the mutual understanding that is needed to agree upon changes appropriate for the community as a whole. In a sense, the novelty of the co-design event itself helped to flatten out some of these inequities: neither the service providers nor the service users had special expertise in co-design, and the process required them to consider how to draw on the different kinds of perspectival expertise (professional, experiential, or both) which they brought to the topic. However, it is also important to note that processes which began during the previous stages of the project had important epistemic 'payoffs' at this point. For example, data collected about all stakeholders' concerns were presented, and weighted equally, to set the agenda for the event. The priorities set during the feedback group discussions were also presented; this is where stakeholders were also invited to consider what the priorities of *other* stakeholders might be, to help to prepare people to work together. Collective involvement (all of the main groups were well-represented) and the visible presence of testimonial evidence at the event meant that the threat of testimonial injustice was greatly diminished at this stage.

Working towards this kind of community involvement may be crucial for supporting the kinds of change which are required. In our project, police participants themselves informed us that they felt that they learned best when they had the opportunity to speak to domestic abuse survivors and perpetrators. Therefore, it may be valuable for the police and the domestic abuse organizations to conduct similar EBCD projects in the future, to be more ambitious in the ways that power is shared, and to develop the capacity to sustain and integrate these ways of working with communities.

In doing so, there is much to be learnt from the expertise of survivor-led movements in other domains, particularly mental health. As other observers have pointed out [12], it is crucial that organizations which draw on the lived experience of their service users make a commitment to acting on what they learn, in order to maintain trust and prevent iatrogenic harms. The degree to which such projects create an opportunity for improving epistemic justice relates directly to the extent to which they are effective, acceptable, and feasible for those they aim to involve, and for those whose experiences they aim to improve.

3.2. Epistemic Justice and Epistemic Capture

In the clustered keypoints which were the focus of our co-design process, participants identified a number of ways in which violence was perpetuated (or went unchecked). We can understand these in relation to the two forms of epistemic injustice. Some work focused implicitly on matters of testimonial injustice (e.g., see the focus of Working Group 1 on the need for more specialist support) and others in relation to hermeneutic injustice in both the short term (e.g., Working Group 4 on improving people's knowledge of when and how to get help) and the long term (e.g., Working Group 4 on educating young people about healthy relational behaviors). Thus, community-based EBCD work *can* be a means of 'building new rooms' [24], in the sense of creating spaces where conversations can take place which do not simply reproduce existing inequalities. In these spaces, collaboration can potentially lead participants down new, more constructive routes. Our experience of conducting EBCD with the police as partners suggests that this *is* possible, but it also highlights some of the ways in which it is difficult.

Police organizations share many features with the health and social care services where EBCD evolved: internal hierarchies, structures linked to budgets, and distinct organizational cultures with preferred ways of controlling and managing change, and preferred ways of identifying and responding to problems, etc. In policing, many of these features are 'writ large' and so the involvement of more vulnerable partners (domestic abuse survivors) comes with the potential for 'epistemic capture' [25].

Epistemic capture refers to the risk that the knowledge produced with and by survivors may be co-opted by more powerful partners, and that survivors have little eventual say in how it is used and acted upon. In contrast, expert-by-experience researchers have argued persuasively that the route to more equitable and effective services lies not in bypassing survivors' ownership of their expertise, but in empowering it [26–28]. To some extent, this highlights a limitation of prevailing models of acceptability [20]. Many dimensions of the acceptability construct resonate with issues we have discussed in this paper. 'Affective attitude,' 'burden,' and 'ethicality' from the Sekhon et al. model [20] seem particularly salient. However, there is a background assumption that interventions come from above, rather than being developed from the bottom up, and it may be that the acceptability concept needs further development to incorporate issues of power and justice, as co-design approaches to intervention become more commonplace.

Initially, this epistemic capture appeared to be the case in our project. After the co-design event, there was little dialogue about the action plans—though there was a commitment made to implementing them. However, previous EBCD researchers have written about the way that co-design processes can be a 'trojan horse' for culture change, promoting improvements to mutual understanding [29] even while stakeholders are ostensibly focused on action-planning. Interestingly, some initiatives which followed in the wake of our project appeared to acknowledge the importance of centering survivors' experiences in determining policy. For example, there was a personal testimony event for survivors which in turn led to a revised policy plan from police commissioners.

Our project relied on those in power to offer opportunities to survivors to share power. Given that opportunity, survivors *did* design action plans alongside service providers during the co-design event. In addition, there was representation of survivors on the steering group, who were involved in the implementation of the project. For example, they provided their feedback on the interview schedule, developed recruitment strategies, reviewed the keypoints, and assisted with planning and running the co-design event. Thus, the co-design approach used in this project tried to encourage citizen participation by creating several platforms in which survivors worked in partnership with their service providers to co-design improved services. This does not flatten the underlying inequalities: service providers could simply decide not to implement the action plans generated from the project, if they wished. From an ethical point of view, it is obviously important that co-design processes lead to change. In our project, the co-design results were incorporated into the regional strategic plan, but as we have discussed, beyond the point of plans and policies, it became difficult to track any changes made. This is a challenge for co-design processes which often involve handover at the implementation stage.

There *are* means by which future EBCD projects could support greater power sharing and epistemic equality in this context. These include paying survivors for their contributions to the project; involving survivors in data collection, as interviewers, and analysis; ensuring that they are involved in the leadership team for the full duration through to implementation. A step up from this would be to support and sustain a community-led EBCD group, in order to maintain an ongoing cycle of EBCD-led service improvements, grounded in local experience and expertise.

3.3. Future Research Directions

The critical next step is evidence about the effectiveness of utilizing EBCD in this setting [20]. To gather this evidence, it is necessary to conduct studies which identify *what changes are made* through the co-designed plans, and which capture how these are achieved. Studies will then be required which can propose and test mechanisms by which those innovations might *reduce violence* and *improve user experience*. It is also clear from the CORE study in Australia [30] that EBCD work can be conducted at scale, across large organizations, and so a further step in terms of feasibility and effectives would involve exploring how parallel EBCD programs might be associated with more diffuse changes in culture and behavior.

4. Conclusions

This project has demonstrated that EBCD can be implemented in a policing setting with victims of crime—particularly with domestic abuse survivors—which can be adopted into police work. Thus, by using EBCD we have the potential to design action plans which improve police services in a manner which listens to the needs of the survivors as well of their service providers. We have also reflected on some implications for police practice as well as on the feasibility and acceptability of such initiatives. We have also suggested potential future research directions which would help examine the acceptability of using an EBCD approach in this context. Since using such an approach has the potential to improve services for domestic abuse survivors and their service providerswe hope that future EBCD projects in a policing setting will be implemented, so that police services can be genuinely co-designed. It is important that such implementations—and their potential effects on survivor well-being, staff workload, complaint reduction, and prosecutions—are tracked, evaluated, and made public. In conclusion, through an EBCD approach in a policing setting, we can potentially make a difference for the people who matter.

Author Contributions: Conceptualization, S.G.-Z., G.L.U., M.L.; methodology, S.G.-Z., G.L.U., M.L.; data collection, S.G.-Z., G.L.U., M.L.; data management, M.L., S.G.-Z.; data analysis, S.G.-Z., G.L.U., M.L.; writing—original draft preparation, S.G.-Z., M.L., G.L.U.; writing—review and editing, S.G.-Z., G.L.U., M.L.; supervision, M.L.; project administration, S.G.-Z., G.L.U., M.L. (with special thanks to the members of the project steering group); funding acquisition, M.L., G.L.U. All authors have read and agreed to the published version of the manuscript.

Funding: This research received partial funding from the regional Police and Crime Commissioner's Office and from the corresponding regional Police Force. S.G.-Z.'s PhD was partially funded through a scholarship from the University of Birmingham.

Institutional Review Board Statement: All research components underpinning the project discussed here were reviewed and approved (ERN15-0752) by the University of Birmingham's Research Ethics Committee.

Informed Consent Statement: Informed consent was obtained from all participants involved in the research components of the project.

Acknowledgments: The authors wish to thank everyone involved with the various stages of the project, including Jessica Woodhams, John Rose, Fay Julal Cnossen, Alex Copello, Amanda Wood, J'Nae Christopher, Shioma-Lei Craythorne, Anna Smith, Lydia Mason and Louise Dixon. We would especially like to thank the survivors and professionals who supported the project, and the members of the steering group (Keith Fraser, Gemma Hickman, Lucy Wright, Kathy Cole-Evans, Harjeet Chakira & Jo Barber).

Conflicts of Interest: The authors declare no conflict of interest.

References

1. World Health Organisation. *Violence against Women Prevalence Estimates, 2018: Global, Regional and National Prevalence Estimates for Intimate Partner Violence against Women and Global and Regional Prevalence Estimates for Non-Partnersexual Violence against Women*; World Health Organization: Geneva, Switzerland, 2021; Licence: CC BY-NC-SA 3.0 IGO.
2. Office for National Statistics. Domestic Abuse in England and Wales Overview: November 2021. Available online: https://www.ons.gov.uk/peoplepopulationandcommunity/crimeandjustice/bulletins/domesticabuseinenglandandwalesoverview/november2021 (accessed on 13 May 2022).
3. Office for National Statistics. Domestic Abuse Prevalence and Trends, England and Wales: Year Ending March 2021. Available online: https://www.ons.gov.uk/peoplepopulationandcommunity/crimeandjustice/articles/domesticabuseprevalenceandtrendsenglandandwales/yearendingmarch2021 (accessed on 13 May 2022).
4. Office for National Statistics. Domestic Abuse Victim Characteristics, England and Wales: Year Ending March 2020. Available online: https://www.ons.gov.uk/peoplepopulationandcommunity/crimeandjustice/articles/domesticabusevictimcharacteristicsenglandandwales/yearendingmarch2020 (accessed on 13 May 2022).
5. Katerndahl, D.; Ferrer, R.; Burge, S.; Becho, J.; Wood, R. Recurrent patterns of daily intimate partner violence and environment. *Nonlinear Dyn. Psychol Life Sci.* **2010**, *14*, 511–524.
6. Liang, B.; Goodman, L.; Tummala-Narra, P.; Weintraub, S. A theoretical framework for understanding help-seeking processes among survivors of intimate partner violence. *Am. J. Community Psychol.* **2005**, *36*, 71–84. [CrossRef] [PubMed]
7. Lelaurain, S.; Graziani, P.; Lo Monaco, G. Intimate Partner Violence and Help-Seeking. *Eur. Psychol.* **2017**, *22*, 263–281. [CrossRef]
8. Fugate, M.; Landis, L.; Riordan, K.; Naureckas, S.; Engel, B. Barriers to domestic violence help seeking: Implications for intervention. *Violence Against Women* **2005**, *11*, 290–310. [CrossRef] [PubMed]
9. SafeLives. Getting It Right First Time. 2015. Available online: https://safelives.org.uk/sites/default/files/resources/Getting%20it%20right%20first%20time%20-%20complete%20report.pdf (accessed on 13 May 2022).
10. Johnson, I.M. Victims' perceptions of police response to domestic violence incidents. *J. Crim. Justice* **2007**, *35*, 498–510. [CrossRef]
11. Bate, P.; Robert, G. *Bringing User Experience to Healthcare Improvement: The Concepts, Methods and Practices of Experience-Based Design*; Radcliffe: Oxford, UK, 2007; 224p.
12. Donetto, S.; Pierri, P.; Tsianakas, V.; Robert, G. Experience-based co-design and healthcare improvement: Realizing participatory design in the public sector. *Des. J.* **2015**, *18*, 227–248. [CrossRef]
13. Donetto, S.; Tsianakas, V.; Robert, G. *Using Experience-Based Co-Design (EBCD) to Improve the Quality of Healthcare: Mapping Where We Are Now and Establishing Future Directions*; King's College London: London, UK, 2014.
14. Mulvale, G.; Moll, S.; Miatello, A.; Robert, G.; Larkin, M.; Palmer, V.J.; Powell, A.; Gable, C.; Girling, M. Co-designing health and other public services with vulnerable and disadvantaged populations: Insights from an international collaboration. *Health Expect.* **2019**, *22*, 284–297. [CrossRef] [PubMed]
15. Dimopoulos-Bick, T.L.; O'Connor, C.; Montgomery, J.; Szanto, T.; Fisher, M.; Sutherland, V.; Baines, H.; Orcher, P.; Stubbs, J.; Maher, L.; et al. "Anyone can co-design?": A case study synthesis of six experience-based co-design (EBCD) projects for healthcare systems improvement in New South Wales, Australia. *Patient Exp. J.* **2019**, *6*, 15. [CrossRef]
16. Division of Cancer Control and Population Sciences (DCCPS). Qualitative Methods in Implementation Science: A White Paper. National Cancer Institute (NIH). 2020. Available online: https://cancercontrol.cancer.gov/sites/default/files/2020-09/nci-dccps-implementationscience-whitepaper.pdf (accessed on 13 May 2022).
17. Fricker, M. *Epistemic Injustice: Power and the Ethics of Knowing*; Oxford University Press: Oxford, UK, 2007.
18. Hänel, H. Who's to Blame? Hermeneutical Misfire, Forward-Looking Responsibility, and Collective Accountability. *Soc. Epistemol.* **2021**, *35*, 173–184. [CrossRef]
19. Mason, E. What Is Hermeneutical Injustice and Who Should We Blame? Social Epistemology Review and Reply Collective. 2021. Available online: https://social-epistemology.com/2021/04/16/what-is-hermeneutical-injustice-and-who-should-we-blame-elinor-mason/ (accessed on 13 May 2022).

20. Sekhon, M.; Cartwright, M.; Francis, J.J. Acceptability of healthcare interventions: An overview of reviews and development of a theoretical framework. *BMC Health Serv. Res.* **2017**, *17*, 88. [CrossRef]
21. Smith, J.A. Semi-structured interviewing and qualitative analysis. In *Rethinking Methods in Psychology*; Smith, J.A., Harre, R., Van Langenhove, L., Eds.; Sage: London, UK, 1995.
22. Barber, J.; Chakira, H.; Cole-Evans, K.; Fraser, K.; Gander-Zaucker, S.; Hickman, G.; Larkin, M.; Unwin, G.; Wright, L. Understanding and Improving the Helpseeking Journey for Survivors of Domestic Abuse. 2018.
23. Stanko, E.A.; Hohl, K. Why Training Is Not Improving the Police Response to Sexual Violence Against Women: A Glimpse into the 'Black Box' of Police Training. In *Women and the Criminal Justice System*; Milne, E., Brennan, K., South, N., Turton, J., Eds.; Palgrave Macmillan: Cham, Switzerland, 2018. [CrossRef]
24. Táíwò, O. Being in the Room Privilege: Elite Capture and Epistemic Deference. *Philosopher* **2020**, *108*, 61–70. Available online: https://www.thephilosopher1923.org/essay-taiwo (accessed on 13 May 2022).
25. Jones, N. Twitter Thread. 2022. Available online: https://twitter.com/viscidula/status/1482393715188580353 (accessed on 13 May 2022).
26. Noorani, T. Service user involvement, authority and the 'expert-by-experience' in mental health. *J. Political Power* **2013**, *6*, 49–68. [CrossRef]
27. Mazanderani, F.; Noorani, T.; Dudhwala, F.; Kamwendo, Z.T. Knowledge, evidence, expertise? The epistemics of experience in contemporary healthcare. *Evid. Policy* **2020**, *16*, 267–284. [CrossRef]
28. Rose, D. Participatory research: Real or imagined. *Soc. Psychiatry Psychiatr. Epidemiol.* **2018**, *53*, 765–771. [CrossRef] [PubMed]
29. Boden, Z.; Springham, N.; Larkin, M. Using experience-based co-design to improve impatient mental health spaces. In *Mental Distress and Space: Community and Clinical Applications*; Reavey, P., McGrath, L., Eds.; Routledge: Oxford, UK, 2017.
30. Palmer, V.J.; Chondros, P.; Piper, D.; Callander, R.; Weavell, W.; Godbee, K.; Potiriadis, M.; Richard, L.; Densely, K.; Herrman, H.; et al. The CORE study protocol: A stepped wedge cluster randomised controlled trial to test a co-design technique to optimise psychosocial recovery outcomes for people affected by mental illness in the community mental health setting. *BMJ Open* **2015**, *5*, e006688. [CrossRef] [PubMed]

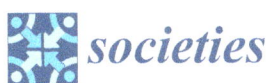

societies

MDPI

Concept Paper

Collaborative Approaches to Addressing Domestic and Sexual Violence among Black and Minority Ethnic Communities in Southampton: A Case Study of Yellow Door

Oluwatayo Adeola Olabanji

DIA and ISVA Services, Yellow Door, Southampton SO17 1QR, UK; oluwatayo.olabanji@yellowdoor.org.uk

Abstract: Domestic and sexual abuse have been in the academic discourse for quite some time. In recent years in the United Kingdom, the government, non-governmental organisations (NGOs) and the charity sector have doubled their efforts to tackle this challenge through different approaches. One of these approaches is the establishment of specialist services. A case study of these specialist interventions is two advocacy services within a community-based domestic and sexual abuse charity in Southampton named Yellow Door (YD). In line with the specialist service approach (SSA), the diversity, inclusion and advocacy (DIA) service and the Black and minority ethnic Communities (BME) independent sexual violence advisory (ISVA) service were created to address the needs of the BME community. Through the adoption of the collaboration, prevention and education approach, these services support survivors from this community, professionals and community groups to encourage more disclosures and support clients holistically. Recommendations to encourage more reporting and better ways to improve the needs of clients from BME communities were proposed.

Keywords: domestic and sexual violence; BME; Yellow Door; prevention; collaborative; education; community-based advocacy

Citation: Olabanji, O.A. Collaborative Approaches to Addressing Domestic and Sexual Violence among Black and Minority Ethnic Communities in Southampton: A Case Study of Yellow Door. *Societies* **2022**, *12*, 165. https://doi.org/10.3390/soc12060165

Academic Editors: Jaimee Mallion and Erika Gebo

Received: 12 October 2022
Accepted: 14 November 2022
Published: 19 November 2022

Publisher's Note: MDPI stays neutral with regard to jurisdictional claims in published maps and institutional affiliations.

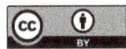
1. Introduction

Violence against women and girls has varied definitions, as it is multi-faceted. However, the definition from the World Health Organisation [1] is the most recognised and globally accepted definition. WHO defines domestic violence as "any act of gender-based violence that results in, or is likely to result in, physical, sexual, or mental harm or suffering to women, including threats of such acts, coercion or arbitrary deprivation of liberty, whether occurring in public or private life". The United Nations [2,3], on the other hand, define domestic violence or abuse "as a pattern of behaviour in any relationship that is used to gain or maintain power and control over an intimate partner," They posit that abuse might be physical, sexual, emotional, economic or psychological actions or threats of actions that influence another person. It further defines sexual violence "as any sexual act, attempt to obtain a sexual act, or other act directed against a person's sexuality using coercion, by any person regardless of their relationship to the victim, in any setting. It includes rape, defined as the physically forced or otherwise coerced penetration of the vulva or anus with a penis, other body part or object, attempted rape, unwanted sexual touching and other non-contact forms" [1]. Domestic abuse, domestic violence or intimate partner violence can be used interchangeably; however, for this conceptual study, the term "domestic abuse" will be adopted. Harmful practices as a subset of violence against women and girls will also be examined.

According to Chan [4], sexual violence is widely acknowledged as a violation of human rights and a public health concern that occurs across societies and cultures, in peace and conflict, and many social settings such as the home, workplace, schools and communities. Unlike the common myth that strangers often perpetrate rape and sexual assaults, statistics show that these crimes are predominantly perpetrated by trusted family members such as partners, cousins, etc. For child sexual abuse (CSA), trusted family or community members, including parents, siblings, and sometimes religious leaders, are often the perpetrators [5]. It is important to state that there are exceptions to this assertion, as this is not always the case.

Supporting the views of [4,6], noted that sexual violence incidents are diverse in circumstances and settings. These could be sexual violence in a romantic relationship, including marriage and dating relationships; rape in non-romantic acquaintances; sexual abuse by those in positions of trust such as clergy, professionals, teachers, medical practitioners, and strangers; multiple perpetrator rapes; sexual trafficking; unwanted sexual contact; and sexual abuse of people with disabilities, among others. These depict the unequal imbalance of relationships between men and women. The keyword in these varied circumstances is consent, which is either not given or not partially given [7]. Notably, although both genders are affected by domestic and sexual violence, women and girls are disproportionately more affected than their male counterparts.

The Home Office shows that one in four women and one in six men have been victims of domestic and sexual abuse in England and Wales. In addition, one in nine or ten women experiences domestic violence in a year [8]. Despite the recent awareness and campaign to increase the inclusion of men in combatting violence against women and girls, statistics show that most domestic abuse victims are women and girls [9]. Women are also more likely to be repeat victims, threatened, harassed, assaulted, and at greater risk of death pre- and post-separation or divorce ([10,11]).

Netto [12], Valente& Wight [13] concluded that domestic and sexual abuse have both damning physical, psychological, and health consequences for the survivors and children in these relationships. Domestic violence survivors often suffer from low self-esteem and mental health issues, and children from these relationships also suffer from physical assault by the same perpetrators [14]. The health implications of sexual violence can range from short- to long-term consequences, including gastrointestinal symptoms, genital injuries and cardiopulmonary symptoms such as palpitations and shortness of breath. Long-term consequences include genital irritation, fibroids, and chronic pelvic pain among others [15].

The aims of this conceptual study is to demonstrate the establishment of specialist services as an example of good practice in the UK; to depict the resultant effects of the establishment of specialist services on disclosures by the BME communities, using Yellow Door as a case study; and to advocate the need for the establishment of more local specialist services away from major cities such as London, Birmingham and Manchester, particularly in locations with a high population in the BME demographic. Finally, this study aimed to re-emphasise the role of collaborative approaches in preventing and reducing domestic abuse and harmful practices. Firstly, this study explains the progress made by charities in post-war Britain in supporting domestic and sexual abuse victims in the United Kingdom; secondly, a brief background of Yellow Door and the two specialist services are discussed; thirdly, BME-specific domestic and sexual abuse will be explained; fourthly, the specialist service approach (SSA) is explored as a framework for collaborative interventions; and lastly, Yellow Door, as a case study of multi-agency collaboration in Southampton, is discussed. Recommendations will be made to facilitate more disclosures and create referral pathways for potential clients.

2. The Role of Charities in Tackling Domestic Violence in Post-War Britain

Domestic violence or abuse was neither in the academic discourse nor incorporated into government policies for a long time in the United Kingdom until very recently (the last three decades). It was considered a private affair that should not be brought to the public domain [16]. The last three decades have seen a significant shift in the understanding, approach and response to domestic violence, nationally and internationally. Governments and international organisations (such as the United Nations and World Health Organisation), and local charities in the UK; specifically, have been instrumental to this shift. For instance, in Britain, 150 years ago, it was legal for a man to beat his wife, provided that he used a stick no thicker than a thumb. Until much attention was given and awareness raised to combat this social problem, no policies or legislation were available to protect domestic violence victims [10].

Since the 1990s, the approach to domestic violence has taken a new outlook, both internationally and locally. This approach is evidenced through several international instruments enacted by international organisations such as the United Nations [17]. The 1995 Fourth World Conference marked a defining moment for the achievement of gender equality, which encapsulated everything gender-related, including violence against women [18]. The Convention on the Elimination of all Forms of Discrimination against Women at the Beijing Conference provided a global framework in which governments from different countries built policies and frameworks for addressing violence against women and girls (VAWG), including domestic and sexual violence [19].

Similarly, the Istanbul Convention, signed in May 2011, emphasised that governments must address all forms of violence against women and girls by condemning this societal problem. The Istanbul Convention defines VAWG "as all forms of violence within the definition experienced by women and girls under 18. This includes domestic violence- all acts of physical, sexual, psychological or economic violence occurring in the family, domestic unit or between current or former spouses or partners" [20]. This definition has been adopted as the standardised framework for both statutory and non-statutory agencies, "which is important for funding, commissioning and multi-agency working" [21].

In the United Kingdom (UK), for instance, feminist policies and movements helped bring the issue of domestic violence to the fore through debates, policymaking and human rights campaigns; a plethora of research attests to this. Subsequently, their campaigns, lobbying and advocacy resulted in the provision of refuges in the 1970s for supporting women who had experienced domestic violence. Due to the massive influx into the refuges, more refuges were established. This influx also birthed Women's Aid and other charities. Other non-governmental organisations have since been established in the UK to cater to domestic and sexual violence victims' needs [22].

According to Harwin [10], "Women's Aid coordinates a national network of 340 local domestic violence services that support more than 500 refuge projects, helplines, and outreach services, including specialist projects for Black and ethnic minority women". The 1980s also saw the establishment of specialist refuges for women of colour and minority communities; these refuges were established following several campaigns by women's organisations to specifically cater to the needs of women from these communities [23,24]. Researchers have further argued that globalisation has been an impetus for the extent and classification of violence against women. More opportunities have been provided for both sexes, including women and girls from all walks of life, as victims of different types of abuse ranging from entrapment, exploitation and abuse to enslavement [22]. Boyle [25] further corroborated the prevalence of violence against women in the UK, stating that "Police reports suggest that domestic violence is a fact of life for millions of women in the UK" [25].

Moving on from the establishment of charities supporting domestic violence victims, domestic and sexual abuse charities have since expanded their thematic areas. From policy advocacies, research focusing on women's separation from their violent spouses or partners, women's welfare benefits such as the Destitution Domestic Violence (DDV) visa housing provision, consultancy, national publicity and training services to emergency protection, the focus of victim support charities have since changed [26]. This activism by these organisations has resulted in tremendous progress, including the domestic abuse act's criminalisation and the domestic abuse bill's passage. This has also increased in the reporting of domestic abuse offences and allegations by 65.8% in London after being reported to the Crime Prosecution Service [10,22].

3. BME, Domestic and Sexual Violence, and Specialist Services

Ethnic minority communities have a migration history with four main ethnicity elements: race, language, culture and religion. These elements differentiate them from their indigenous Anglo-Saxon counterparts in the United Kingdom. These factors should be considered when supporting members of these communities [27,28]. Siddiqui [29] argued that the high rate of domestic and sexual abuse among BME could be attributed to the more significant barriers they face due to intersectional discrimination based on factors such as race, class, caste, poverty overlaps and other multiples. Graca [30] further stated that women from these communities face additional barriers, such as insecure immigration status. In addition, the socio-cultural practices of non-UK nationals compared with other counterparts impede them from accessing support services.

Martin, Jahan & Habib [31] opine that Asian women face double abuse, as they are often victimised first by the abuser and the community. The responsibility of protecting the family honour ("Izzat" in Urdu) and the avoidance of bringing shame ("Sharam" in Urdu) to the family debar women from these communities from escaping domestic and sexual abuse [32]. Since communities are commonly complicit in these hidden crimes, fear of reprisals from the community silence many women and girls from reporting [33]. The study by Mulvihill, Walker, Hester & Gangoli [34] identified that religion is adopted as a manipulative tool by both families and religious organisations to convince women from BME backgrounds to remain in abusive relationships. These foundations stem from religious texts which justify women's reasons to only leave a marriage on the grounds of death or infidelity [35]. Conversely, in Islam, men can divorce a woman by saying the word "talaq" three times, which gives men a kind of coercive control in an abusive relationship and makes women perpetual victims [36].

Netto [12] explored an underreported barrier to reporting in the BME communities. She argued that this is based on the importance of honour attached to the family. Some women from these communities have internalised the feeling of inferiority to their male counterparts in the family and, as such, feel responsible for the different forms of abuse, such as the physical, emotional and sexual abuse they experience from family members and in-laws. Some of these barriers sometimes hinder them from leaving abusive relationships and seeking professional support.

However, Ahmed [37] differs in his findings, as he concludes that Black and minority ethnic communities come from a wide range of varied backgrounds, including religious, cultural [38] and socio-economic backgrounds, compared with other communities. As such, different services should be provided for these communities that are different from the mainstream communities. Chand &Thoburn [39] further observed a shortage of preventative work, specialist services and service delivery for children and families from Black and minority ethnic communities across the UK. VAWG [21] arrived at a somewhat different conclusion. Their research concluded that specialist services, particularly community-based women's organisations, are pivotal to the prevention of and intervention in VAWG. Their conclusion is due to the familiarity with the local terrain and their ability to build a framework around education, innovation and prevention. Larasi [26] further stressed that due to the knowledge of the local communities, the establishment of specialist services for Black and minoritized women and girls are critical. These services provide advocacy and frontline responses alongside campaigning and lobbying at the national front, which, in turn, translate into positive outcomes such as more disclosures, holistic support and rebuilding their lives after the abuse.

Despite the proliferation of women's groups and organisations supporting women experiencing domestic abuse and the increase in the reporting of domestic abuse among Black and minority ethnic communities, evidential research has shown underreporting or no reporting at all for women experiencing domestic and sexual abuse in the BME communities exists [40]. Specific vulnerabilities such as insecure immigration status [41], cultural and religious factors, and policies and structures such as having no recourse to public funds are the principal factors contributing to the underreporting of domestic violence within these communities [42].

Gangoli, Bates,& Hester [43] argued that the most common type of abuse experienced and reported by BME women was all-encompassing abuse and different from other communities. In addition to physical, financial, sexual and emotional abuse experienced by other communities, some members from the BME communities further experience other harmful practices such as honour-based abuse, forced marriages, breast flattening, and Female Genital Mutilation(FGM), among others [44]. They are, thus, faced with a two-edged sword of abuse. It was further observed that compared with their White British counterparts, the disclosure rate of sexual-related offences experienced by both adults and children from BME groups was low due to the culture of "shame" linked to issues around rape and assault [45]. Dartnall & Jewkes [6] attributed the underreporting of domestic and sexual violence among the BME community to factors such as having fewer specialist services, a lack of awareness of specialist services, cultural and religious barriers, immigration status and the different legal and cultural requirements in their home countries [43].

The End Violence against Women Coalition remarked on the dearth of research into the impact of specialist services on the reporting and disclosure of domestic and sexual abuse among BME communities [46]. They further highlighted how the nature of the cultural advocacy and support provided impacts domestic and sexual disclosures and reporting. Hence, the need to investigate this research gap. There is less emphasis on programmes focusing on preventative work and education of BME communities and the long-term consequences of domestic and sexual abuse on their members. Solutions to tackle this problem within the community are also missing [47].

4. Yellow Door—A Brief Background and Two Specialist Services

Yellow Door (YD) is a domestic and sexual abuse charity established 36 years ago as a rape crisis service in Southampton, United Kingdom. Since its inception, it has expanded to provide a range of prevention and support interventions to victims of domestic abuse and other forms of interpersonal harm or discrimination.

Yellow Door is an inclusive charity that works with any gender and all age groups. It also supports victims of domestic and sexual abuse in whatever form, at whatever stage or form of life, regardless of the time, historical or recent.

Most of the services provided by Yellow Door are from the central premises in Southampton or Southampton in general; other services are, however, provided across some areas in Hampshire, depending on funding availability.

Yellow Door provides domestic and sexual abuse support through six different services, namely therapeutic services, domestic abuse services, independent sexual violence advisory services (ISVA), diversity and inclusion advocacy (DIA), the helpline, and prevention and education [48].

In addition, to specifically cater to the needs of the Black, Asian and minority ethnic (BAME) communities within Southampton, a bridged service between the diversity and inclusion services and the independent sexual violence advisors service was created. This research focused on this bridged service between the ISVA and DIA services, catering to the domestic and sexual concerns of the victims and survivors from these communities. For context, the terms BAME or BME will be briefly explained to understand this demographic. BAME or BME represents the Black, Asian and minority ethnic communities or those with BME (Black and minority ethnic) backgrounds. To better support clients from these backgrounds with additional needs and specific vulnerabilities, YD collaborates with other statutory and non-statutory agencies across Southampton and Hampshire to provide them with holistic support.

4.1. Yellow Door Specialist Services—ISVA/DIA Services

4.1.1. The Independent Sexual Violence Advisory Service (ISVA)

Both the DIA and ISVA services within YD use the empowerment or client-led approach, building on evidential research of its effectiveness to provide holistic support to clients [49]. The empowerment-oriented approach is predicated on the two social work principles of "self-determination and the dignity and worth of human beings". This approach postulates that clients should be involved in decision-making regarding their service delivery and have access to quality holistic services best suited to their needs and well-being [50]. These empower clients, help them develop leadership skills and increase self-esteem [51]. The independent sexual violence advisory service (ISVA) is an advocacy service within Yellow Door that specialises in supporting victims of any unwanted sexual experience such as sexual violence, abuse or exploitation, regardless of the incident, whether historical or recent, and regardless of age, gender or sexuality. The providers are professionally trained to provide personalised emotional and practical support to meet clients' needs. Although they work closely with the police, they are an independent service that provides independent support to help clients make informed decisions about their next steps [52].

ISVAs provide support with decisions, reporting to the police and health options, and support throughout the criminal justice process, depending on the client's choice or decision. Specialist services include the children and young persons' ISVA, the family ISVA, the male ISVA and the BAME ISVA within the ISVA services. This research, however, focuses on the BAME ISVA specialist service [52].

4.1.2. BAME ISVA

BAME ISVA workers are specialists who support clients from Black and minority ethnic communities who have suffered sexual abuse, exploitation and violence across Hampshire. The BAME independent sexual violence advisory service within YD supports sexual violence victims, from the reporting to the investigation stage, and throughout the criminal justice process.

According to YD, below is a table and chart showing the ISVA service users' demographics (Table 1 and Figure 1).

Table 1. ISVA service users' demographics: Number of service users accessing the ISVA service from October 2021 to September 2022.

ISVA Service Users' Demographics: Number of Service Users Accessing the ISVA Service				
	October–December Q3 2021/2022	January–March Q4 2021/2022	April–June Q1 2022/2023	July–September Q2 2022 3
White (English, Welsh, Scottish, Northern Irish, Irish, any other White background)	84	299	341	262
BME (White European/other, mixed/multiple ethnic groups, Asian/Asian British (including Chinese, Indian, Pakistani, Bangladeshi and any other Asian background), Black/African/Caribbean/Black British, other ethnic group (including Arab and any other ethnic groups) and Gypsy/Traveller)	6	39	37	31
Not stated	19	127	160	93
Total	109	465	538	386

The table above shows the number of service users per year from October 2021 to September 2022.

The third quarter shows a total of 109 service users: 84 White clients, 6 BME clients and 19 not stated. The last quarter in 2021/2022, between January to March 2022, saw a massive increase of 299 service users. This increase marked a milestone for the BME ISVA services, as the number increased from 6 in the last quarter to 39. This massive increase in service users can be attributed to the BBC report [53], which stated that violence against women in Hampshire increased significantly in 2022. Southampton, Portsmouth and Basingstoke saw a rise in sexual violence cases, Southampton being the highest, with a total of 402. The increase in BME clients can also be attributed to the establishment of the BME specialist service in September 2021.

The first quarter of 2022/2023 saw a slight increase in service users, totalling 341 White clients, 37 BME clients and 160 not stated. The second quarter of 2022/2023 saw a relative decline in White, BME and "not stated" clients, with 262, 31 and 93, respectively.

Although the number of BME service users was low compared with their White British counterparts, the progress and increase are noteworthy, considering the barriers mentioned above experienced by this demographic. It is essential to consider that the number of those in the "not stated" category was huge in all the quarters. Although not accounted for, one can infer that BME clients are also within these numbers. Nevertheless, it is safe to conclude that the establishment of the BME ISVA service translated into an increased number of disclosures and, in turn, service users from that community.

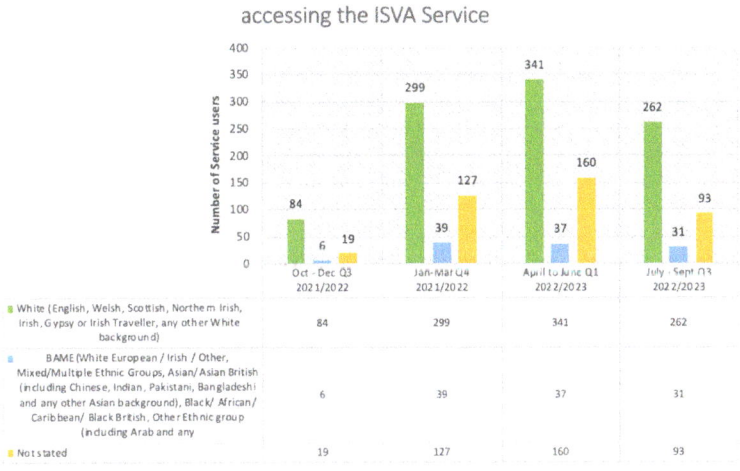

Figure 1. ISVA service users' demographics: number of service users accessing the ISVA service.

Figure 1 illustrates the graphical representation of Table 1.

4.2. The Diversity and Inclusion Advocacy Service (DIA)

This advocacy service within YD includes domestic and sexual abuse specialists trained to work with marginalised or disadvantaged groups or communities to address barriers, such as language, ethnicity, disability, sexuality, faith, and mental health to improve access and promote equality. Professionals within this service speak multiple languages, such as South Asian, African and European, to support and address language barriers among the minority ethnic communities they support. There are also specialist services within this service.

4.2.1. Harmful Practices

The harmful practices workers or advocates (HPWs) provide emotional and practical support to the victims or those at risk of harmful practices such as female genital mutilation (FGM), forced marriage, honour-based abuse and breast flattening. These specialists also support clients with complex needs and specific vulnerabilities, such as housing, immigration status and education, through one-to-one casework [52].

4.2.2. Prevention and Education

To tackle the recurrence of domestic and sexual abuse, mainly hidden harm, the HPWs within the DIA service engage in educational sessions in primary and secondary schools in Southampton. They educate children, young people and undergraduates on harmful practices such as FGM, forced marriage, honour-based abuse and breast flattening.

These specialists also work collaboratively with other professionals in Hampshire, the Isle of Wight, Portsmouth and Southampton (HIPS) to run webinars on HP for the police, social services, tertiary sector, education and health professionals to identify the risks and create referral pathways for clients.

4.2.3. Training

The HPW practitioners design training packages for professionals, taking factors such as the specific sector, the audience, the best-suited safeguarding protocols and relevant terminologies into consideration when delivering this training to designated safeguarding leads (DSLs), headteachers and other leads in education settings. Training and webinars are also delivered to other professionals in the health sector, including general practitioners (GPs) and midwives.

Both the ISVA and DIA services provide emotional and practical support to survivors from this community. They also raise awareness in different communities and religious organisations to encourage more disclosures and reporting. Both services also work collaboratively with other institutions, professionals and community-based organisations such as the police, the criminal justice system, Early Help, the Southampton City council and other charities in Southampton, among others.

5. Specialist Service Approach: A Multi-Agency Framework

Logar & Vargová [54] defined specialist or women's support services as a collection of specialist services covering a range of thematic areas in supporting the victims and survivors of domestic violence. These thematic areas ranging from women's shelters, national women's helplines, rape crisis and sexual assault referral centres, migrant and minority ethnic women, and independent domestic and sexual violence advocacy to intervention centres. The multi-agency approach is considered effective for preventative and early intervention in domestic abuse services at both the operational and strategic levels, resulting in holistic support, effective service delivery and positive outcomes for the service's users [55]. For instance, at Yellow Door, to safeguard a domestic violence victim living with the perpetrator whose life is at risk, the best practice is to secure a safe space for the client by either signposting the victim to a women's refuge or seeking alternative accommodation. This safeguarding is achieved by collaborating with the local police, housing practitioners and refuges across the country to protect the victim. This is, of course, achieved with the client's consent.

Cheminais [56] provided some benefits of collaborative or multi-agency partnerships in the education sector, which also apply to other professional settings. The benefits range from "enhanced and improved outcomes for children and young people through ease of access, and support, strengthening partnership, breaking down professional boundaries and parochial attitudes, to building consensus". Atkinson et al. [57] also argued that the multi-agency helps to build a more cohesive community approach through the practitioners taking greater ownership and responsibility for addressing local needs jointly, thus avoiding duplication or overlap of provision.

In Southampton's violence against women and girls sector, the multi-agency approach entails working collaboratively with the police, the criminal justice system, the witness service and other local charities with different thematic areas.

Though there are different models available to be adopted, there are, three broad models a multi-agency framework can use in executing its functions. While some use the expertise of practitioners who meet regularly, some adopt the casework method, while others engage designated workers to lead the casework [58]. Atkinson et al. [57] differed somewhat in their description of the multi-agency approach, arguing that there are five different "multi-agency models: decision-making groups, consultation and training, centre-based delivery, coordinated delivery, and operational-team delivery". They further opined that different organisations or agencies adopt different models and meet for varied reasons to achieve a primary purpose or objective.

The three models described above by [58] are adopted at Yellow Door, depending on the client's circumstances. A case in point of using the expertise of practitioners who meet regularly to support a client is the Multi-Agency Risk Assessment Conference (MARAC) meeting. This meeting is where different professionals discuss relevant information, safe-guarding and potential support. These professionals could be local police, health, children's services, housing practitioners, independent domestic violence advisor (IDVAs), independent sexual violence advisors (ISVAs) and other practitioners to protect the highest-risk domestic violence victims.

The casework approach is another method adopted by YD, as BAME ISVAs and harmful practices workers provide one-to-one casework support to the victims of harmful practices and sexual violence. ISVAs, for instance, support clients from the pre-reporting stage and throughout the police investigation to the trial and post-trial stages, unless otherwise requested by the client. Designated workers with specific expertise also support clients within the purview of their expertise. BAME ISVAs support BAME clients, whereas children's ISVAs support child clients. This approach is used to achieve tailored support. In the case of victims of HP, only the HPWs equipped with the right expertise are designated to support these clients. The HPWs are also active stakeholders in the HP operational group and the FGM Zero Tolerance Day in Southampton.

6. Yellow Door and Multi-Agency Collaboration in Southampton

Collaborative working in combating domestic and sexual abuse requires sufficient funding, alongside a strong partnership among statutory services such as the police, housing, health services, the Crown prosecution service, the criminal justice system, children's and social services, and commissioners, among others [59]. Non-statutory agencies such as charities with similar thematic areas but different jurisdictions are also pivotal in providing holistic care and support for clients and survivors. These factors are also considered the basis of local funding for local organisations [21]. Some organisations and institutions involved in the collaborative efforts in different ways with Yellow Door in Southampton, United Kingdom, are described below.

6.1. The Police

The police support different areas of DV, ranging from honour-based abuse, domestic abuse, female genital mutilation, and breast flattening, among others. For instance, Yellow Door and the police co-chair the Harmful Practices Operational Group. YD also works closely with the Chief Inspector, including partnering on the FGM Crime Stoppers initiative and engaging with police constables to reach communities.

Similarly, within the police is a special unit called "Amberstone". They are specially trained officers (also known as STOs) who have been specially trained to support sexual violence victims from the reporting to the investigation stage.

6.2. Specially Trained Officers (STOs)

The STOs are also called sexual offences investigative techniques trained officers (SOIT officers), depending on the county or police force involved. STOs are responsible for providing clients with practical and emotional support throughout the investigation process. Some of the primary responsibilities of the STOs are to take the victim's initial report of the incident and statement and signpost clients to the relevant agencies, including sexual violence specialist services such as the independent sexual violence advisory service. STOs also ensure that the medical needs of sexual violence victims are met; this is accomplished by referring clients to sexual assault referral centres. They educate clients on the criminal justice system, provide relevant information regarding the case and safeguard clients at risk. For clients contemplating reporting, YD works collaboratively with the STOs to provide "Anonymous Advice Meetings", where the clients meet with the STOs in a relaxed environment to gain clarity about the criminal justice process and to decide their next steps [60].

6.3. Sexual Assault Referral Centres

The sexual assault referral centres (SARC) are medical sexual violence health centres across the nation targeted at anyone who has experienced sexual violence. They provide medical treatment and forensic medical examinations. The SARC is a 24 h service and a collaboration between the police, the National Health Services and charities. SARC referrals can be made by specially trained police officers or ISVA services, or victims of sexual violence can report the incident independently without the involvement of the police. Forensic examinations in these centres can be kept for a while, regardless of the decision to report or not [60].

6.4. Southampton City Council

Within Southampton City Council, a team of professionals is dedicated to supporting high-risk clients who may be victims of VAWG, such as domestic abuse, honour-based abuse, forced marriage, female genital mutilation and sexual violence. The Multi-Agency Safeguarding Hub (MASH) in Southampton provides "triage and multi-agency assessment of safeguarding concerns" [61] This team protects the most vulnerable children and adults from harm, neglect and abuse by meeting goals related explicitly to safeguarding [61]. The purpose is to respond quickly to safeguarding concerns about vulnerable children. It also aims at partnerships, collaborative communication and reducing inappropriate referrals and re-referrals. MASH referrals are often sent from YD to the local authority to protect and support vulnerable children, adults and families to ensure holistic support.

6.5. Other Agencies

YD adopts a "Coordinated Community Response (CCR), a coordinated response aimed at reforming, improving and coordinating institutional responses to domestic violence within the community" to support clients holistically [54]. Thus, YD collaborates with other community-based statutory and non-statutory agencies to support the needs of clients outside the jurisdiction of Yellow Door. Some of these services and institutions are The University of Southampton, Early Help, general practitioners (GPs), midwives, the police and housing for the DIA service. Witness care and witness services within the Crown prosecution service, also work closely with the ISVA service.

Despite these collaborations, both services encounter some challenges when delivering services. For instance, the DIA service's one-to-one advocacy support, was impacted by COVID-19, as the clients' movements were restricted. The service adopted Zoom sessions during this period and has continued to adapt to hybrid working modes. In addition to HP, some of our clients have multiple vulnerabilities, such as learning disabilities, visual impairments, hearing difficulties, etc. Due to these added complexities, engaging via telephone or Zoom could be logistically challenging. The HPWs adapt to the challenge of medium and location continually.

Another major challenge is the language barrier. Some of our service users have limited command of the English language, thus making support a challenge. The HPWs speak European, South Asian and African languages that are well suited to the clientele. In the event of the non-availability of some languages, the HPWs use certified interpreters to support clients.

Disclosures of forced marriages and honour-based abuse often result in some clients seeking alternative accommodation separate from the perpetrators. The HPWs mitigate this housing challenge by working collaboratively with the police and refuge workers to provide temporary accommodation in refuges. The HPWs also work closely with housing officers to provide permanent accommodation as required.

With respect to the BME ISVA service, one of the foremost challenges is the long duration of the criminal justice process, which sometimes discourages clients from reporting or results in the withdrawal of cases. The BME ISVAs confront this by managing clients' expectations from the outset through anonymous advice meetings. Expectations and outcome are also managed through one-to-one support of the clients throughout the investigative process. Unfavourable trial and post-trial outcomes can also sometimes negatively impact or traumatise clients. Signposting clients to the appropriate trauma-informed service and counselling services within and outside Yellow Door often tackles this challenge.

7. Discussion

According to the British Broadcasting Corporation [53], violence against women in Hampshire and the Isle of Wight increased to 37,137 offences in 2021. Rape incidents in 2021 increased to 402 in Southampton, with the highest rate; one in six rapes in Hampshire was committed in Southampton. They also observed that Southampton, Portsmouth and Basingstoke have higher numbers of other sexual offences. Hence, the need to establish additional domestic and sexual abuse specialist services to address these challenges in Hampshire and across the United Kingdom. Yellow Door, a community-based domestic and sexual abuse charity in Southampton, has been addressing these societal concerns by establishing varied services addressing specific domestic and sexual-related concerns and issues. YD has seen a 91% increase in referrals, with Southampton ranking as the second-highest city for sexual offences in England, and the figure has increased by 240% in the last five years [48]. Thus, YD and various agencies must continue to work collaboratively to combat this challenge and make the city safer for women and girls to reside in.

Disclosures among the BME communities are challenging because of the factors mentioned above. Some clients within these communities have also experienced mistrust from service providers in the past, thereby leading to dire consequences from family and community members.

1. Establishing more specialist services serve as a safe space for supporting BME victims and survivors. The establishment of more specialist services for Black and minority ethnic communities in more local areas across the United Kingdom will cater to their specific needs and encourage more disclosures and reporting of domestic and sexual abuse in these communities.

2. Increasing long-term funding for existing specialist services will result in the continuity of these services, as clients will be confident that their needs will be addressed long-term. This approach will potentially reduce the observed underreporting of domestic and sexual abuse within these communities.

3. Thus, to provide more opportunities for disclosures, more specialist services should be established to safeguard the clients and ensure that the client's trust is gained. The assurance of confidentiality in handling their cases is also critical, as disclosures could potentially result in honour-based abuse by families and community members.

4. More advocacy strategies are required to incorporate more community stakeholders such as clergy and local community leaders in the combat against domestic and sexual abuse among BME. These stakeholders are critical to effecting the desired change of

eliminating domestic and sexual violence within the BME communities and in the United Kingdom.

5. Increased training on cultural competence for statutory and non-statutory professionals such as the police, local authorities and other practitioners should be advocated. This training will ensure that clients from these communities feel confident and safe enough to disclose cases and are also assured of non-judgmental or stereotypical interventions by professionals.

6. More specialist refuges or women's shelters specific to the BME communities should be established across the country to cater to the specific needs of this demographic of clients. These shelters will serve as safe spaces and safeguard victims from perpetrators.

7. The four crucial peculiarities of BME clients: race, culture, language and religion, should always be considered whilst providing interventions for these clients' demographics. Considering these factors will ensure the provision of holistic support.

8. Conclusions

This research has highlighted the collaborative approaches to addressing domestic and sexual abuse among the Black and minority communities in Southampton, England, using two specialist services within Yellow Door as case studies. The need for specialist services for minority ethnic groups to better cater to their needs based on their specific vulnerabilities was discussed. Factors such as immigration status, language barriers, religion, honour-based abuse and other vulnerabilities which differ from the mainstream community, were also considered.

Yellow Door's multi-agency approach with statutory and non-statutory organisations across Southampton to support the varied and complex needs of clients from Black and minority ethnic communities through various strategies such as prevention and education was also highlighted. This research has observed the effectiveness of the specialist service approach, from a practitioner's standpoint. Unlike in the past, where domestic and sexual abuse in Southampton and Western Hampshire within the Black and minority ethnic communities was underreported, both specialist services within YD have seen more referrals from professionals and community groups. Self-referrals from survivors regarding both historical and recent sexual abuse have also been observed. Disclosures of harmful practices such as forced marriage, honour-based abuse and female genital mutilation have also increased in these communities.

Clients have also attested to the effectiveness of the casework interventions received from both services, resulting in improved mental and physical well-being. Thus, it is safe to say that establishing specialist services for Black and minority ethnic communities translates into more disclosures and reporting by these communities, and specialist casework interventions promote improved well-being.

Funding: This research received no external funding.

Institutional Review Board Statement: Not applicable.

Informed Consent Statement: Not applicable.

Data Availability Statement: Data are not public according to ethical guidelines.

Conflicts of Interest: The author declares no conflict of interest.

References

1. World Health Organization. Violence Against Women. 2021. Available online: https://www.who.int/news-room/fact-sheets/detail/violence-against-women (accessed on 27 September 2022).
2. UN. What Is Domestic Abuse? 2020. Available online: https://www.un.org/en/coronavirus/what-is-domestic-abuse (accessed on 11 November 2022).
3. Walklate, S.; Godfrey, B.; Richardson, J. Changes and continuities in police responses to domestic abuse in England and Wales during the COVID-19 'lockdown'. *Polic. Soc.* **2022**, *32*, 221–233. [CrossRef]

4. Chan, K.L. Sexual Violence Against Women and Children in Chinese Societies. *Trauma Violence Abus.* **2009**, *10*, 69–85. [CrossRef] [PubMed]

5. Tishelman, A.C.; Fontes, L.A. Religion in child sexual abuse forensic interviews. *Child Abuse Negl.* **2017**, *63*, 120–130. [CrossRef]

6. Dartnall, E.; Jewkes, R. Sexual violence against women: The scope of the problem. *Best Pract. Res. Clin. Obstet. Gynaecol.* **2013**, *27*, 3–13. [CrossRef] [PubMed]

7. Gill, A. 'Crimes of Honour' and Violence against Women in the UK. *Int. J. Comp. Appl. Crim. Justice* **2008**, *32*, 243–263. [CrossRef]

8. Home Office. Domestic Abuse: How to Get Help. 2012. Available online: https://www.gov.uk/guidance/domestic-abuse-how-to-get-help (accessed on 11 November 2022).

9. Itzin, C.; Taket, A.R.; Barter-Godfrey, S. (Eds.) *Domestic and Sexual Violence and Abuse: Tackling the Health and Mental Health Effects;* 1. publ.; Routledge: London, UK, 2010.

10. Harwin, N. Putting a Stop to Domestic Violence in the United Kingdom: Challenges and Opportunities. *Violence Women* **2006**, *12*, 556–567. [CrossRef]

11. Lloyd, M.; Ramon, S. Smoke and Mirrors: U.K. Newspaper Representations of Intimate Partner Domestic Violence. *Violence Women* **2016**, *23*, 114–139. [CrossRef] [PubMed]

12. Netto, G. Vulnerability to Homelessness, Use of Services and Homelessness Prevention in Black and Minority Ethnic Communities. *Hous. Stud.* **2006**, *21*, 581–601. [CrossRef]

13. Valente, S.; Wight, C. Military Sexual Trauma: Violence and Sexual Abuse. *Mil. Med.* **2007**, *172*, 259–265. [CrossRef]

14. Rakovec-Felser, Z. Domestic violence and abuse in intimate relationship from public health perspective. *Health Psychol. Res.* **2014**, *2*, 1821. [CrossRef]

15. Priester, M.A.; Cole, T.; Lynch, S.M.; DeHart, D.D. Consequences and Sequelae of Violence and Victimization. In *The Wiley Handbook on the Psychology of Violence;* Cuevas, C.A., Rennison, C.M., Eds.; John Wiley & Sons, Ltd.: Chichester, UK, 2016; pp. 100–119. [CrossRef]

16. Kelly, J.B.; Johnson, M.P. Differentiation Among Types of Intimate Partner Violence: Research Update and Implications for Interventions. *Fam. Court Rev.* **2008**, *46*, 476–499. [CrossRef]

17. Krook, M.L.; True, J. Rethinking the life cycles of international norms: The United Nations and the global promotion of gender equality. *Eur. J. Int. Relations* **2012**, *18*, 103–127. [CrossRef]

18. Chant, S. The 'Feminisation of Poverty' and the 'Feminisation' of Anti-Poverty Programmes: Room for Revision? *J. Dev. Stud.* **2008**, *44*, 165–197. [CrossRef]

19. United Nations Human Rights Office of the High Commissioner. Committee on the Elimination of Discrimination against Women. 2022. Available online: https://www.ohchr.org/en/treaty-bodies/cedaw (accessed on 10 September 2022).

20. Niemi-Kiesiläinen, J.; Peroni, L.; Stoyanova, V. (Eds.) *International Law and Violence Against Women: Europe and the Istanbul Convention;* Milton Park: Abingdon, Oxon, UK; Routledge: New York, NY, USA, 2020.

21. VAWG. Joint Principles for the VAWG Strategy 2021–2024. *The Government's Call for Evidence for the Next VAWG Strategy for 2021–2024.* 2021. Available online: https://irisi.org/wp-content/uploads/2021/02/Joint-Principles-for-the-VAWG-Strategy-2021-2024.pdf (accessed on 27 September 2022).

22. Radford, L.; Tsutsumi, K. Globalization and violence against women—Inequalities in risks, responsibilities and blame in the Uk and Japan. *Women's Stud. Int. Forum* **2004**, *27*, 1–12. [CrossRef]

23. Thiara, R. Strengthening diversity: Response to BME women experiencing domestic violence in the UK. In Proceedings of the European Conference on Interpersonal Violence, Paris, France, 26 September 2005; Volume 2005.

24. Anitha, S. Neither safety nor justice: The UK government response to domestic violence against immigrant women. *J. Soc. Welf. Fam. Law* **2008**, *30*, 189–202. [CrossRef]

25. Boyle, A. Incidence and prevalence of domestic violence in a UK emergency department. *Emerg. Med. J.* **2003**, *20*, 438–442. [CrossRef]

26. Larasi, M. A fuss about nothing? Delivering services to black and minority ethnic survivors of gender violence: The role of the specialist black and minority ethnic women's sector. In *Moving in the Shadows: Violence in the Lives of Minority Women and Children,* 1st ed.; Routledge: London, UK, 2013; pp. 276–282.

27. Kelly, L. *Moving in the Shadows: Violence in the Lives of Minority Women and Children,* 1st ed.; Routledge: London, UK, 2016. [CrossRef]

28. Sawrikar, P.; Katz, I. Proposing a Model of Service Delivery for Victims/Survivors of Child Sexual Abuse (CSA) from Ethnic Minority Communities in Australia. *J. Soc. Serv. Res.* **2018**, *44*, 730–748. [CrossRef]

29. Siddiqui, S. *Trump Administration Moves to End Asylum for Victims of Domestic Abuse and Gangs;* Wash. Post: Washington, DC, USA, 2018.

30. Graca, S. Domestic violence policy and legislation in the UK: A discussion of immigrant women's vulnerabilities. *Eur. J. Curr. Leg. Issues* **2017**, *22*, 1–34.

31. Martin, J.; Jahan, N.; Habib, T. *Sisters against Abuse (SAA).* 2020. Available online: https://thetrf.org/wp-content/uploads/2020/06/SAA-final-report.pdf (accessed on 10 September 2022).

32. Chantler, K.; Gangoli, G. *Violence against Women in Minoritised Communities: Cultural Norm or Cultural Anomaly?* Verlag Barbara Budrich. Social Science Open Access Repository: Opladen, Leverkusen, Germany, 2011.

33. Fleming, K.; Kruger, L. "She keeps his secrets": A gendered analysis of the impact of shame on the non-disclosure of sexual violence in one low-income South African community. *Afr. Saf. Promot. J. Inj. Violence Prev.* **2013**, *11*, 107–124.
34. Mulvihill, N.; Walker, S.-J.; Hester, M.; Gangoli, G. *How Is 'justice' Understood, Sought, and Experienced by Victims/Survivors of Gender-Based Violence? A Review of the Literature*; University of Bristol: Bristol, UK, 2018.
35. Witte, J. *From Sacrament to Contract: Marriage, Religion, and Law in the Western Tradition*, 2nd ed.; Westminster John Knox Press: Louisville, KY , USA, 2012. [CrossRef]
36. Hidayat, I.; Yaswirman, Y.; Mardenis, M. Problems Arising from Talak Divorce Outside the Court. *Int. J. Multicult. Multireligious Underst.* **2019**, *6*, 138–148. [CrossRef]
37. Ahmed, S. What is the Evidence of Early Intervention, Preventative Services for Black and Minority Ethnic Group Children and their Families? *Practice* **2005**, *17*, 89–102. [CrossRef]
38. Lockhart, L.L.; Danis, F.S. *Domestic Violence: Intersectionality and Culturally Competent Practice*; Columbia University Press: New York, NY, USA, 2010.
39. Chand, A.; Thoburn, J. Research Review: Child and family support services with minority ethnic families: What can we learn from research? *Child Htmlent Glyphamp Asciiamp Fam. Soc. Work* **2005**, *10*, 169–178. [CrossRef]
40. Belur, J. Is policing domestic violence institutionally racist? A case study of south Asian Women. *Polic. Soc.* **2008**, *18*, 426–444. [CrossRef]
41. Safe Lives. *Safe Lives Calls for Government to Allocate Adequate Funding to Support Migrant Survivors of Domestic Abuse with Insecure Immigration Status*. 2022. Available online: https://safelives.org.uk/funding-to-support-migrant-survivors (accessed on 10 September 2022).
42. Anitha, S. Legislating Gender Inequalities: The Nature and Patterns of Domestic Violence Experienced by South Asian Women with Insecure Immigration Status in the United Kingdom. *Violence Women* **2011**, *17*, 1260–1285. [CrossRef]
43. Gangoli, G.; Bates, L.; Hester, M. What does justice mean to black and minority ethnic (BME) victims/survivors of gender-based violence? *J. Ethn. Migr. Stud.* **2020**, *46*, 3119–3135. [CrossRef]
44. Gill, A.K.; Walker, S. On Honour, Culture and Violence Against Women in Black and Minority Ethnic Communities. In *The Emerald Handbook of Feminism, Criminology and Social Change*; Walklate, S., Fitz-Gibbon, K., Maher, J., McCulloch, J., Eds.; Emerald Publishing Limited: Bingley, UK, 2020; pp. 157–176. [CrossRef]
45. Cowburn, M.; Gill, A.K.; Harrison, K. Speaking about sexual abuse in British South Asian communities: Offenders, victims and the challenges of shame and reintegration. *J. Sex. Aggress.* **2015**, *21*, 4–15. [CrossRef]
46. Coy, M.; Kelly, L.; Foord, J.; Bowstead, J. Roads to Nowhere? Mapping Violence Against Women Services. *Violence Women* **2011**, *17*, 404–425. [CrossRef]
47. Coalition, E.V.A.W. *Attitudes to Sexual Consent*; End Violence Against Women: London, UK, 2020.
48. Yellowdoor. Yellowdoor: Who We Are. 2022. Available online: https://yellowdoor.org.uk/about-us/ (accessed on 27 September 2022).
49. Hardina, D. *An Empowering Approach to Managing Social Service Organizations*; Springer: New York, NY, USA, 2007.
50. Hardina, D. Ten Characteristics of Empowerment-Oriented Social Service Organizations. *Adm. Soc. Work* **2005**, *29*, 23–42. [CrossRef]
51. Hardina, D.; Montana, S. Empowering Staff and Clients: Comparing Preferences for Management Models by the Professional Degrees Held by Organization Administrators. *Soc. Work* **2011**, *56*, 247–257. [CrossRef]
52. Yellowdoor. Independent Sexual Violence Advisors (ISVA). 2022. Available online: https://yellowdoor.org.uk/services/isva-service/ (accessed on 27 September 2022).
53. BBC South. 2022. Available online: https://www.bbc.co.uk/programmes/b006pfl4 (accessed on 10 September 2022).
54. Logar, R.; Vargová, B. *Effective Multi-Agency Co-Operation for Preventing and Combating Domestic Violence Training of Trainers Manual, 2015*; Council of Europe: Strasbourg, France, 2021.
55. Cleaver, K.; Maras, P.; Oram, C.; McCallum, K. A review of UK based multi-agency approaches to early intervention in domestic abuse: Lessons to be learnt from existing evaluation studies. *Aggress. Violent Behav.* **2019**, *46*, 140–155. [CrossRef]
56. Cheminais, C. The Origin, Concept and Principles of Multi Agency Partnership Working. In *Effective Multi-Agency Partnerships: Putting Every Child Matters into Practice*; SAGE Publications Ltd.: London, UK, 2008; pp. 1–22.
57. Atkinson, M.; Wilkin, A.; Scott, A.; Doherty, P.; Kinder, K. *Multi-Agency Work: A Detailed Study*; National Foundation for Educational Research: Berkshire, UK, 2002.
58. Workingham. Fact Sheet. Multi-Agency Working. 2005. Available online: https://www.wokingham.gov.uk/EasysiteWeb/getresource.axd?AssetID=75433& (accessed on 27 September 2022).
59. Coy, M.; Kelly, L.; Foord, J.; Balding, V.; Davenport, R. Map of gaps: The postcode lottery of violence against women support services. In *End Violence Against Women*; End Violence Against Women: London, UK, 2007.
60. Rightofwomen. From Report to Court a handbook for Adult Survivors of Sexual Violence. 2014. Available online: https://rightsofwomen.org.uk/wp-content/uploads/2016/11/From-Report-to-Court-a-handbook-for-adult-survivors-of-sexual-violence.pdf (accessed on 10 September 2022).
61. Southampton City Council. The Children's Resource Service. 2022. Available online: https://www.southampton.gov.uk/health-social-care/children/child-social-care/childrens-resource-service/ (accessed on 21 October 2022).

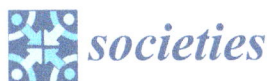

societies

MDPI

Article

Reflections on Increasing the Value of Data on Sexual Violence Incidents against Children to Better Prevent and Respond to Sexual Offending in Kenya

Zidan Ji [1], Sarah Rockowitz [2], Heather D. Flowe [2], Laura M. Stevens [2], Wangu Kanja [3] and Kari Davies [4,*]

[1] Institution of Education, University College London, London WC1E 6BT, UK; zidan.ji.19@alumni.ucl.ac.uk
[2] School of Psychology, University of Birmingham, Birmingham B15 2TT, UK;
sxr1005@student.bham.ac.uk (S.R.); h.flowe@bham.ac.uk (H.D.F.); lms825@student.bham.ac.uk (L.M.S.)
[3] Wangu Kanja Foundation, Nairobi 12608, Kenya; wangukanja@gmail.com
[4] Department of Psychology, Bournemouth University, Poole BH12 5BB, UK
* Correspondence: kadavies@bournemouth.ac.uk

Abstract: In many countries, data collection on sexual violence incidents is not integrated into the healthcare system, which makes it difficult to establish the nature of sexual offences in this country. This contributes to widespread societal denial about the realities of sexual violence cases and the collective oppression of survivors and their families. Capturing detailed information about incidents (e.g., characteristics of perpetrators, where it happened, victims, and the offence) can dispel myths about sexual violence and aid in crime prevention and interventions. This article examines how information about sexual violence incidents—in particular, offences committed against children in Kenya—is gathered from two different data sources: the Violence Against Children Survey (VACS) and data collected by the Wangu Kanja Foundation (WKF), a survivor-led Kenyan NGO that assists sexual violence survivors in attaining vital services and justice. These two surveys provide the most comprehensive information about sexual and gender-based violence. The analysis indicates that, while the VACS provides information about the prevalence of sexual violence, it provides less detailed information about the nature of violence (e.g., characteristics of perpetrators, victims, and the offence) compared with the WKF dataset. We critically reflect on how validity and informativeness can be maximised in future surveys to better understand the nature of sexual violence, as well as other forms of gender-based violence, and aid in prevention and response interventions/programming.

Keywords: sexual violence; child sexual violence; survey data; data collection; gender-based violence

Citation: Ji, Z.; Rockowitz, S.; Flowe, H.D.; Stevens, L.M.; Kanja, W.; Davies, K. Reflections on Increasing the Value of Data on Sexual Violence Incidents against Children to Better Prevent and Respond to Sexual Offending in Kenya. *Societies* **2022**, *12*, 89. https://doi.org/10.3390/soc12030089

Academic Editors: Jaimee Mallion and Erika Gebo

Received: 21 February 2022
Accepted: 25 May 2022
Published: 6 June 2022

Publisher's Note: MDPI stays neutral with regard to jurisdictional claims in published maps and institutional affiliations.

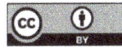
1. Introduction

Sexual violence is a human rights and public health issue of concern worldwide and is defined as the use of coercion by any person in any situation to experience a sexual act. Sexual violence includes rape, attempted rape, unwanted sexual contact, and other non-contact offences [1]. It is one of the world's most widespread non-communicable diseases and human-rights abuses [2,3]. Some factors around the world that are associated with the perpetration of sexual violence include beliefs about sexual purity and family honour, patriarchal societies, the acceptability of violence against women, and weak legal punishments for sexual violence [1]. The 2014 Kenya Demographic and Health Survey (KDHS) indicated that approximately 45% of women and girls between the ages of 14 and 49 have been subjected to some form of violence, with 14% subjected to sexual violence [4]. In addition, sexual violence is frequently not reported to the police, and offenders are seldom arrested, let alone prosecuted [5,6]. Furthermore, victims are often held accountable for the offence, even by the organisations responsible for serving and protecting survivors (e.g., the police) [7].

The aim of this paper is to critically discuss the types of data that are needed to improve our understanding of the nature of sexual violence in low- and middle- income countries, and in Kenya in particular. Kenya is a country that has a growing national grassroots network of sexual violence survivors that assists victims and advocates for policy and practice change nationally. Like in many countries, survivors in Kenya struggle to access vital services (e.g., emergency medical care, safe shelters), and prosecutions are extremely rare. We consider data held by the Survivors of Sexual Violence in Kenya Network (hereafter, the Network), a grassroots survivor-led community organisation that has been gathering data about sexual violence and other violations. These data on violations against children can help us to better understand the types of offences that are occurring, the vital services that are needed, and the causes of case attrition along the case referral pathway when survivors seek vital support.

A key driver of sexual violence, which predominantly affects women and children, is gender inequality: Kenya ranks 142 out of 189 countries on the Gender Equality Index, with 11 million women in Kenya experiencing sexual and/or physical violence during their lifetime [8,9]. Compounding this, in Kenya, survivors face overly bureaucratic and poorly resourced systems that are laced with corruption, and they are often fearful of reprisal by perpetrators and discouraged by non-empathetic responses from law enforcement [10]. Survivors also face stigma from their communities and families. The impact of sexual violence itself, coupled with the poor societal response to sexual violence, negatively impacts the survivor's health, the development of their children, and the economic and social attainment of their families; thus, cycles of violence and pain continue, and multiple, layered, and even simultaneous experiences of violence persist into future generations, creating new challenges and blocking change [2,11–13].

Sexual violence affects people in Kenya starting at a young age and is a daily reality [14]. This occurs partly because violence is often used as a means of conflict resolution. Patriarchal ideals reinforce male social power, and violence is exacerbated by the widespread issue of poverty and low educational attainment. Additionally, victims of all ages are discouraged from reporting their cases to the authorities in Kenya. This, coupled with resource constraints, means that children often do not have access to justice [14]. A significant portion of the Kenyan population is children, with 40% of Kenyans being under the age of 18; 250,000 of these children live on the street [14]. Throughout the country, children face barriers to educational attainment. Some geographic regions have student– teacher ratios of 77 to 1 [15]. Dropout is also a significant issue, especially in pastoral communities [15]. Financial and resource constraints also lead to dropout. Many girls must miss school to fetch wood or water for their families, others are forced to miss days due to menstrual hygiene management issues, and still, others are pulled out of school to be married off, which leads to further violence [16].

The Kenyan legal framework prohibits violence against children. An early regulation pertaining to violence against children is the Children and Young Person Act of 1964. It penalises anyone responsible for assaulting, mistreating, neglecting, or abandoning children (or exposing them to any of these acts) aged 0 to 16 years [14]. The act was expanded in 2002 to grant rights to children, including rights to education, protection from harmful cultural rites, healthcare, and protection from child labour and armed conflict, as well as rights to protection from sexual abuse and exploitation [14]. The act was again revised in 2012 to include provisions that afford children protection from abuse and neglect, both physical and psychological, female circumcision and other cultural rites that may be harmful, sexual exploitation, and torture or cruel treatment [17]. The Sexual Offences Act was passed in 2006, and it provides definitions of child sexual abuse, such as prohibiting sexual contact with girls under the age of 16 who are unmarried and boys before the age of 12, and prohibits incest, defilement, trafficking, and forced marriage [18]. The term 'defilement' describes an act that causes the penetration of a child younger than age 18. Punishment varies depending on the age of the child. Defilement of a child younger than age 11 can carry a term of life imprisonment, whereas defilement of a child who is 12 to 15 years old carries a minimum of 20 years imprisonment and defiling a child who is 16 to 18 years old carries a sentence of at least 15 years imprisonment [19].

Much of our knowledge about sexual violence and other forms of violations against children is based on the results of the Violence Against Children Survey (VACS), which is a UNICEF- and CDC-backed national survey that has been administered in various countries around the world, including Kenya, Rwanda, Lao PDR, and Uganda. The VACS is the main, if not the only, source of systematic data about sexual violence in many countries. For example, in the US, data about sexual offences are compiled across law enforcement agencies nationally via the Uniform Crime Reports and gathered via national victim surveys. Comparable data sources are not available in Kenya. However, national data on child sexual violence are critically important for developing, financing, and coordinating national prevention and response strategies; the next section provides an overview of how the VACS is conducted, along with an analysis of some of its key strengths and limitations, followed by a discussion of the ways in which data could be improved to help prevent child sexual violence in Kenya.

2. The Violence against Children Survey (VACS)

The VACS is administered periodically over so many years as a cross-sectional house-hold survey throughout Kenya. The survey collects information about the national prevalence of violence and seeks to identify risk and protective factors, health consequences, and public knowledge of services. The VACS is conducted via collaborations between international aid organisations and local government bodies, such as the Ministry of Education and the National Bureau of Statistics. Kenya's 2010 VACS was the country's first national survey of violence against male and female children [20]. The VACS collects information on current and lifetime experiences of sexual, physical, and emotional violence for children, who are divided into two age groups: 13- to 17-year-olds and 18- to 24-year-olds. The 13- to 17-year-olds are asked about their experiences with violence during the 12-month period prior to their taking the survey, whereas the 18- to 24-year-olds are asked about their life experiences with violence [20]. The administrators choose households from different communities around Kenya based on randomly selected clusters, and then different areas are assigned as either male or female survey spots. This is to ensure the confidentiality of respondents' data, as well as to prevent male perpetrators and female victims from the same community both being interviewed in case the perpetrator finds out about the intention of the study and chooses to retaliate against their victim(s) for taking part [20]. Desired sample sizes for each sex were determined by using data from the Kenya Demographic Health Survey (DHS) to estimate the proportion of households with residents of the desired age and sex group [20].

The VACS interview process consists of a brief demographic interview with the head of the household, followed by a comprehensive interview of the household members, including questions about the respondent's experiences of having violence inflicted on them as a child [20]. The questions included in the survey were developed based on questions from other international and national surveys, such as the DHS, HIV/AIDS surveys, the WHO Multi-country Study on Women's Health and Domestic Violence Against Women, etc. [20]. Thirty-two teams with three-to-five interviewers and one team leader each collected data throughout the country, all supervised by coordinators from the Kenya National Bureau of Statistics and technical advisors from the CDC in the US [20]. Questions on the survey cover physical, sexual, and emotional violence for both sexes in both age groups. Physical violence includes being slapped, kicked, whipped, beaten with an object, pushed, punched, threatened, or attacked with a weapon [20]. Sexual violence includes unwanted touching in a sexual way, unwanted attempted intercourse, pressured intercourse, and physically forced intercourse. Finally, emotional violence includes being humiliated on purpose, made to feel unwanted, or threatened with abandonment [20]. The survey also collects information on the perpetrator's relationship to the victim, the location and time of day of sexual violence incidents, help-seeking experiences, services received, health outcomes, etc. [20].

The 2010 VACS found that lifetime experiences of sexual violence prior to age 18 were reported by 32% of female respondents and 18% of male respondents aged 18 to 24 [20]. Lifetime physical violence was reported by 66% of females and 73% of males surveyed from the same age group [20]. Current levels of violence, defined as having experienced violence in the 12 months prior to the survey being administered, were also high; specifically, 11% of females and 4% of males aged 13 to 17 reported having experienced sexual violence in the previous 12 months, and 49% of females and 48% of males from the same group reported having experienced physical violence. While the VACS does not include information about the experiences of children who are younger than the age of 13, other studies have found that the most prominent age group for males to experience violence is 0 to 10 years old, and for females, it is 21 to 30 years old [21]. The Kenya DHS collects somewhat similar data on violence, although it focuses more on the adult population. Of note, however, is a question on the DHS that asks about the respondent's first experience of violence, including physical, sexual, or both types of violence. The question asks male and female respondents if they had endured their first experience of sexual violence at different ages, starting at 10 years old, then 12, 15, 18, and 22 [22]. The DHS does not ask who the perpetrators were of this first experience of violence, nor does it ask about help-seeking behaviour or the location of the incident. It also does not explain why these ages were chosen to measure the first experience of violence.

While the VACS provides important data on the national prevalence of different forms of violence experienced by children, there are limitations. First, neither the VACS nor the DHS survey children under the age of 13, or their parents, about life experiences with violence. Furthermore, the VACS does not gather in-depth information about incidents, such as the number of perpetrators involved, whether a weapon was used, whether and how the victim was injured, or whether the victim was alcohol-intoxicated, for example. This type of information can provide details about the perpetrator's behaviour that can aid in crime detection and prevention, such as by uncovering the perpetrator *modus operandi* for purposes of linking crimes committed by serial offenders [23]. Furthermore, the VACS does not provide information about the reporting of incidents to the police, or adjudication, which would allow for studying case attrition, such as identifying regions in which few reported cases are prosecuted. Finally, some of the information being reported by survivors in the VACS concerns incidents of violence that occurred long ago. When testimony about an event is taken relatively recently after the incident, it will be a more complete account [24].

To address knowledge gaps concerning sexual offences committed against children, information might be sourced alternatively from records held by the police, the judiciary, or the NGOs that assist survivors. Information from police and court records, assuming it was made available for research purposes, would provide an incomplete picture of sexual offences. First, few cases are reported to the police, and even fewer lead to a prosecution [25]. Second, while research on the characteristics of adjudicated cases in Kenya is lacking, research from other countries indicates that the characteristics of cases that are prosecuted differ from those that are not [26]. For instance, cases that fit with the 'real rape stereotype' (e.g., the offender is a stranger, the victim is severely injured and reports promptly) are more likely to be reported by victims and accepted by officials for prosecution. What is more, the characteristics of most of sexual offences differ markedly from the real rape stereotype. Consequently, the analysis of cases in which the perpetrator has been identified, arrested, prosecuted, and/or convicted provides a narrow and incomplete understanding of the sexual offending and, thus, has limited utility with respect to informing crime prevention and response strategies across the range of offenses that occur. Furthermore, in investigating and prosecuting sexual violence cases, medico-forensic evidence (e.g., anogenital injury) figures prominently in Kenya, and relatively little information is gathered from survivors about what they remember about the perpetrator and the incident itself [11]. However, the survivor's testimony is indispensable for building a detailed understanding of the offences, as well as of how to prevent and respond to these crimes.

3. Community Data to Address the Limitations of the VACS

Against the backdrop of challenges faced by survivors seeking vital assistance and justice, the Network was established. It was born out of a national survivor-led movement in Kenya and established by the Wangu Kanja Foundation (WKF), a 15-year-old registered non-profit NGO that assists survivors in accessing post-rape care services [27]. The WKF was founded by Wangu Kanja, a rape survivor. The WKF supports adult and child survivors free of charge as they try to access services in Nairobi, the largest criminal jurisdiction in Kenya. The WKF is in Nairobi's Mukuru Kwa Reuben, one of the largest informal settlements in Kenya. It has a population of about 500,000 and a high rate of sexual violence. While many WKF clients are from Mukuru, they also come from surrounding counties. Victims learn about the WKF via radio advertisements and other media and contact WKF via walk-in or SMS, who will then support and accompany both adult and child survivors as they attempt to access services. For each client, the WKF collects data about case progression across the case referral pathway, gathering information about the offence, the victim, and the perpetrator(s), as well as about medical services the client can access, criminal investigation, and case adjudication.

In the next section, we provide an overview of the information being gathered by the WKF, and how it can be used to fill critical gaps in knowledge about sexual and other forms of violence committed against children. While we focus on children, our observations apply to offences committed against adults. We also discuss how collecting more detailed information from survivors about offenses on a routine basis throughout the country would enhance the knowledge base and assist in national efforts to prevent and respond to sexual and other forms of gender-based violence in Kenya, as well as in other countries.

4. A Community Approach to Information Gathering

Table 1 provides a summary of information about sexual violence gathered by the VACS and WKF. One of the most striking differences between the VACS and the data gathered by the WKF and Network concerns the extent to which detailed information is gathered about incidents. The VACS is designed to investigate the prevalence of different forms of violence in relation to age. The survivor's family circumstances, and socio-economic status are recorded in detail, as well as the survivor's attitudes towards help-seeking behaviour. Previous research has shown that children from low-income households are at higher risk of violence [28]; therefore, the household's economic status is important to gather.

In contrast, the WKF collects critical case-related information about the injuries suffered by survivors, as well as data on whether survivors received legal aid, retained forensic evidence, and if so, what it was, and whether the survivor accessed medical and police services. As previously mentioned, the lack of legal aid and timely access to medical and police assistance reduces the likelihood that medico-forensic evidence is recovered. The lack of such evidence is a major cause of case attrition [29]. Consequently, the WKF and Network data can provide valuable information about what evidence is most frequently gathered, and what evidence is most often lacking, which can provide leads about what services are needed to strengthen evidence and prosecutions.

The WKF and Network also record information about survivors' experiences as they negotiate the case referral pathway. Detailed information is obtained about the survivors' ability to access security (e.g., safe houses), medical attention, and police services, as well as information about whether the police documented the case and whether it was ultimately accepted for prosecution. Information about the survivors' medical status in relation to the violation, such as HIV test results, is recorded, unlike the VACS, which can provide information about whether survivors are able to access vital services in the aftermath of sexual violence.

Table 1. Items collected by the WKF compared with the VACS survey.

	Item	WKF	VACS
Demographic Information	Age	✔	✔
	Gender	✔	✔
	Location	✔	✔
	Marital Status		✔
	Education Status		✔
Incident Information	Relationship with Perpetrator	✔	✔
	Attack Location	✔	✔
	Attack Date	✔	
	Attack Time	✔	✔
	Injury Detailed	✔	
Service Access Information	HIV Test and Status	✔	
	Pregnancy Test and Status	✔	✔
	Forensic Evidence	✔	
	Seeking Medical Service	✔	✔
	Seeking Police or Legal Service	✔	
	Seeking Counselling Service	✔	✔
	Court Case Filed	✔	

The WKF and Network take a survivor-focused approach in gathering information from survivors; the community members gathering the information are trained human rights defenders, who are all survivors of sexual violence themselves. They assist the survivors in accessing services and conduct follow-up interviews about the status of the case and the services received. This is not necessarily the case for interviewers who collect data for the VACS.

One key example that demonstrates the value of the types of detailed data being gathered in real time by the WKF and Network concerns the data they collected about violations occurring against children during the COVID-19 pandemic [30–32]. The Network, which operates in all 47 counties in Kenya, continued to assist survivors during periods in which strict curfews were in place. The curfews created obstacles for survivors in accessing vital services and reporting crimes to the police. The data collected indicated that child survivors of sexual and other forms of violence were younger compared to pre-pandemic periods and that children were particularly likely to be violated during the day and by a neighbour [30–32]. In many cases, the neighbour gained access to the child by inviting them to their house under the guise of helping the child access the internet for home-schooling purposes.

The WKF and Network currently also have research underway that is investigating how to improve the quality of the data they are gathering about incidents using questioning techniques that focus on the behaviour of the offender. The research builds the capacity of those gathering data to ask questions that establish the behaviour (i.e., *modus operandi*) of the offender before, during, and after the offence. Behavioural techniques establish how the offender behaved during the offence, including how and where they initially approached the victim, how they maintained control over the victim, and how they left the scene of the crime. These techniques can be useful in at least two ways. First, behavioural information can help to create a more accurate picture of offending and dispel rape stereotypes about offences committed by perpetrators who are strangers as well as known to the victim. As noted above, a 'real rape stereotype' exists wherein sexual violence is only believed to be 'real' if certain behaviours were exhibited (e.g., rape is committed by strangers, using a weapon, and victims physically resist). In reality, sexual violence often does not fit this stereotype, but the persistence of the idea of a 'real rape' means that the veracity or severity of survivors' stories can be downplayed or the survivors themselves can face blame for the offence [5]. Understanding in more detail the true picture of sexual violence in Kenya can provide support for survivors where the offences perpetrated against them deviate from this stereotype. Second, behavioural information can also be used to bolster investigative capacity, helping law enforcement, NGOs, and human rights defenders identify links between offences to highlight where serial offenders may be operating. This behavioural linking of crimes can be particularly useful in cases where no forensic evidence has been collected, or where it is too costly to process [33], but it does require a detailed level of behavioural information for this type of analysis to be conducted. In the Global North and in South Africa, this approach is supported by research [33–37], and such research provides a unique opportunity to document the 'who, what, when, where, and how' of stranger sexual offences [38] in Kenya. In addition to being of urgent relevance to partners and law enforcement stakeholders, the research will bring new insights to the sparse academic literature on the situational crime prevention of sexual offences [39], especially in low-resource contexts where criminal investigation infrastructure is lacking. The research currently being conducted by the WKF and the Network in collaboration the Rights for Time Network (www.rights4time.com, accessed on 20 February 2022) is investigating how behavioural information can be used in Kenya to understand the nature of the offences occurring and to solve crimes.

The survivor-centred approach to gathering data can also increase the willingness of survivors to report incidents that do not conform to the above-mentioned stereotyped views about what constitutes rape. For instance, survivors who were alcohol-intoxicated during the offence or who are acquainted with the offender may be more inclined to report information about their ordeal to the WKF and the Network than they are to VACS or DHS interviewers. Data about incidents of sexual violence in all its forms can serve to counter stereotypes about victims and decrease the stigma and blame that survivors encounter when reporting their cases to the authorities. Furthermore, the WKF and Network use trauma-informed methods to gather information and are trained in the essentials of interviewing techniques. This training is important considering that previous research has found that survivors were more willing to disclose sexual violence when a trauma-informed approach had been utilised [40]. The WKF and Network also function within their communities to raise awareness about what constitutes sexual violence, and this facilitates the reporting of incidents that survivors may not have otherwise realised were legal violations.

There are other key differences in the methodology employed by the VACS and WKF and Network that give rise to unique limitations of both types of surveys that future research must address. A strength of the WKF survey methodology is that it collects information prospectively from survivors in real time, as the case is progressing through the medico-legal system. In contrast, survivors retrospectively report incidents that occurred in the past on the VACS and DHS. The VACS and DHS also do not gather detailed intelligence about survivors' ability to access services. The WKF data, however, do not allow for inferences about the prevalence of sexual violence either within a region or nationally, as the data are gathered using convenience sampling rather than random sampling. To address the limitations of existing surveys, a national monitoring system should be put into place to routinely record information about incidents. Such a system could gather location-specific information to identify crime hotspots where additional security measures are needed to prevent violence, and where increased medical, police, and judicial service provision is necessary to respond to crimes. The system could also potentially assist survivors with reporting their cases to the authorities. Most medical facilities in Kenya do not have forensic laboratories, let alone the post-rape medical care forms required by the police to file charges [41].

Finally, the distressing nature of sexual and other forms of violence means that it is costly for survivors to disclose these incidents, particularly during police interviews. Some studies have shown, for instance, that the willingness of survivors to provide information to investigators is highly correlated with the costs (e.g., re-traumatisation, stigmatisation, etc.) survivors incur in providing that information [42]. However, it usually takes days to weeks for survivors to report a case and receive the necessary forms to complete, and they often need to have the means and time to visit more than one government-designated location/institution for medical examination. The process discourages survivors from engaging with the medico-legal system and re-traumatises and stigmatises them [11]. Initiatives that seek to gather information about sexual violence incidents from survivors need a strong and clear rationale for obtaining the information. Furthermore, the benefits to survivors arising from them disclosing information need to be at the forefront.

5. Conclusions

The aim of this article was to explore how a community approach to gathering detailed information about sexual violence incidents can provide a more comprehensive understanding of sexual offending against children in Kenya. Our research highlights that when collecting information about sensitive and distressing topics such as sexual violence, a key consideration is *how* the data are collected. The methods used to gather data impact the types of incidents that are disclosed. Different methods of data collection can affect (1) people's willingness to disclose incidents in the first place and (2) the accuracy and type of information they divulge [40]. As noted above, the WKF and Network members who gather data from survivors are also survivors of sexual violence and are trusted members of the survivor's local community. As such, this approach increases the willingness of survivors to disclose incidents and provide in-depth information about these assaults that can help increase knowledge about the violations that are occurring to better prevent and respond to crimes in the future.

Author Contributions: Conceptualisation, Z.J., H.D.F. and K.D.; writing—original draft preparation, Z.J., S.R., H.D.F., L.M.S. and K.D.; writing—review and editing, Z.J., S.R., H.D.F., L.M.S., W.K. and K.D.; supervision, K.D. and H.D.F. All authors have read and agreed to the published version of the manuscript.

Funding: This research was supported by the Economic and Social Research Council ES/T010207/1 and the Arts and Humanities Research Council AH/T008091/1.

Institutional Review Board Statement: Not applicable.

Informed Consent Statement: Not applicable.

Data Availability Statement: Not applicable.

Conflicts of Interest: The authors declare no conflict of interest.

References

1. World Health Organization. Violence against Women. 2021. Available online: https://www.who.int/news-room/fact-sheets/detail/violence-against-women (accessed on 30 July 2021).
2. Garcia-Moreno, C.; Jansen, H.A.F.M.; Ellsberg, M.; Heise, L.; Watts, C. *WHO Multi-Country Study on Women's Health and Domestic Violence against Women: Initial Results on Prevalence, Health Outcomes, and Women's Responses*; World Health Organization: Geneva, Switzerland, 2005.
3. Tulchinsky, T.H.; Varavikova, E.A. *The New Public Health*, 3rd ed.; Elsevier: Amsterdam, The Netherlands, 2014.
4. Kenya National Bureau of Statistics and ICF Macro. *Kenya Demographic and Health Survey 2008–09*; KNBS and ICF Macro: Calverton, MD, USA, 2010.
5. Gerd, B.; Friederike, E.; Afroditi, P.; Frank, S.; Tendayi, V. Rape myth acceptance: Cognitive, affective, and behavioural effects of beliefs that blame the victim and exonerate the perpetrator. In *Rape: Challenging Contemporary Thinking*; Taylor Francis Group: Abingdon, UK, 2019. [CrossRef]
6. Brown, J.; Hamilton, C.; O'Neill, D. Characteristics associated with rape attrition and the role played by scepticism or legal rationality by investigators and prosecutors. *Psychol. Crime Law* **2007**, *13*, 355–370. [CrossRef]
7. Seelinger, K. Domestic accountability for sexual violence: The potential of specialized units in Kenya, Liberia, Sierra Leone and Uganda. *Int. Rev. Red Cross* **2014**, *96*, 539–564. [CrossRef]

8. United Nations Development Programme. *Gender Inequality Index*; UN: New York, NY, USA, 2019.
9. National Gender and Equality Commission. National Monitoring and Evaluation Framework towards the Prevention of and Response to Sexual and Gender Based Violence in Kenya. 2014. Available online: https://www.ngeckenya.org/Downloads/National-ME-Framework-towards-the-Prevention-Response-to-SGBV-in-Kenya.pdf (accessed on 20 February 2022).
10. Ondicho, T.G. Violence against Women in Kenya: A Public Health Problem. *Int. J. Dev. Sustain.* **2018**, *7*, 2030–2047. Available online: https://www.researchgate.net/ (accessed on 20 February 2022).
11. Shako, K.; Kalsi, M. Forensic observations and recommendations on sexual and gender based violence in Kenya. *Forensic Sci. Int. Synerg.* **2019**, *1*, 185–203. [CrossRef] [PubMed]
12. World Health Organization. *Global and Regional Estimates of Violence against Women: Prevalence and Health Effects of Intimate Partner Violence and Non-Partner Sexual Violence*; World Health Organization: Geneva, Switzerland, 2013.
13. World Health Organization. *Global Plan of Action to Strengthen the Role of the Health System within a National Multisectoral Response to Address Interpersonal Violence, in Particular against Women and Girls, and against Children*; World Health Organization: Geneva, Switzerland, 2016.
14. Bridgewater, G. Physical and Sexual Violence against Children in Kenya within a Cultural Context. *Community Pract.* **2016**, *89*, 30–34. Available online: https://pubmed.ncbi.nlm.nih.gov/27164800/ (accessed on 20 February 2022).
15. UNICEF. Situation Analysis of Children and Women in Kenya 2017. *Nairobi, Kenya.* 2018. Available online: https://www.unicef.org/kenya/media/136/file/SITAN-report-2017-pdf.pdf (accessed on 20 February 2022).
16. Warrington, M.; Kiragu, S. "It makes more sense to educate a boy": Girls 'against the odds' in Kajiado, Kenya. *Int. J. Educ. Dev.* **2012**, *32*, 301–309. [CrossRef]
17. National Council for Law Reporting. Children's Act. Revised Edition 2012 (2010). 2012. Available online: http://kenyalaw.org/kl/fileadmin/pdfdownloads/Acts/ChildrenAct_No8of2001.pdf (accessed on 20 February 2022).
18. Plummer, C.; Njuguna, W. Cultural protective and risk factors: Professional perspectives about child sexual abuse in Kenya. *Child Abus. Negl.* **2009**, *33*, 524–532. [CrossRef] [PubMed]
19. National Council for Law Reporting. Sexual Offences Act. 2006. Available online: http://kenyalaw.org/kl/index.php?id=1894 (accessed on 20 February 2022).
20. VACS. Violence against Children in Kenya: Findings from a 2010 National Survey. Nairobi, Kenya. 2012. Available online: https://resourcecentre.savethechildren.net/document/violence-against-children-kenya-findings-2010-national-survey-summary-report-prevalence/ (accessed on 20 February 2022).
21. Ongeti, K.; Ogeng'o, J.; Were, C.; Gakara, C.; Pulei, A. Pattern of Gender Based Violence in Nairobi, Kenya. *Int. Res. Med. Sci.* **2013**, *1*, 30–34. Available online: uonbi.ac.ke (accessed on 20 February 2022).
22. DHS. The DHS Program. 2014. Available online: https://dhsprogram.com/ (accessed on 20 February 2022).
23. Woodhams, J.; Bennell, C. (Eds.) *Crime Linkage: Theory, Research, and Practice*, 1st ed.; Routledge: Abingdon, UK, 2014. [CrossRef]
24. Stevens, L.M.; Reid, E.; Kanja, W.; Rockowitz, S.; Davies, K.; Dosanjh, S.; Flowe, H.D. The Kenyan survivors of sexual violence network: Preserving memory evidence with a bespoke mobile application to increase access to vital services and justice. *Societies* **2022**, *12*, 12. [CrossRef]
25. Wangamati, C.K.; Sundby, J.; Izugbara, C.; Nyambedha, E.O.; Prince, R.J. Challenges in supporting survivors of child sexual abuse in Kenya: A qualitative study of government and non-governmental organizations. *J. Interpers. Violence* **2021**, *36*, 15–16. [CrossRef]
26. Patterson, D. The impact of detectives' manner of questioning on rape victims' disclosure. *Violence Against Women* **2011**, *17*, 1349–1373. [CrossRef] [PubMed]
27. WKF. About WKF. 2016. Available online: https://wangukanjafoundation.org/?page_id=2 (accessed on 20 February 2022).
28. Miller, G.; Chiang, L.; Hollis, N. Economics and violence against children, findings from the Violence Against Children Survey in Nigeria. *Child Abus. Negl.* **2018**, *85*, 9–16. [CrossRef] [PubMed]
29. Chamlee, V. These Detroit Rape Kit Statistics Could Mean There Are 29,000 Unknown Serial Rapists in the U.S. 2017. Available online: https://www.bustle.com/p/these-detroit-rape-kit-statistics-could-mean-there-are-29000-unknown-serial-rapists-in-the-us-7638521 (accessed on 21 August 2021).
30. Flowe, H.D.; Rockowitz, S.; Rockey, J.; Kanja, W.; Kamau, C.; Colloff, C.; Kauldar, J.; Woodhams, J.; Davies, K. Sexual and Other Forms of Violence during the COVID-19 Pandemic Emergency in Kenya. 2020. Available online: https://zenodo.cern.ch/record/3964124/files/Covid%20Kenya%20Report_compressed.pdf (accessed on 20 February 2022).
31. Rockowitz, S.; Stevens, L.M.; Rockey, J.C.; Smith, L.L.; Ritchie, J.; Colloff, M.F.; Flowe, H.D. Patterns of sexual violence against adults and children during the COVID-19 pandemic in Kenya: A prospective cross-sectional study. *BMJ Open* **2021**, *11*, e048636. [CrossRef] [PubMed]
32. Stevens, L.M.; Rockey, J.C.; Rockowitz, S.R.; Kanja, W.; Colloff, M.F.; Flowe, H.D. Children's vulnerability to sexual violence during COVID-19 in Kenya: Recommendations for the future. *Front. Glob. Womens Health* **2021**, *2*, 7. [CrossRef] [PubMed]
33. Pakkanen, T.; Sirén, J.; Zappalà, A.; Jern, P.; Bosco, D.; Berti, A.; Santtila, P. Linking serial homicide—Towards an ecologically valid application. *J. Criminol. Res. Policy Pract.* **2021**, *7*, 18–33. [CrossRef]
34. Slater, C.; Woodhams, J.; Hamilton-Giachritsis, C. Testing the assumptions of crime linkage with stranger sex offenses: A more ecologically-valid study. *J. Police Crim. Psychol.* **2015**, *30*, 261–273. [CrossRef]

35. Tonkin, M.; Santtila, P.; Bull, R. The linking of burglary crimes using offender behaviour: Testing research cross-nationally and exploring methodology. *Leg. Criminol. Psychol.* **2012**, *17*, 276–293. [CrossRef]
36. Woodhams, J.; Tonkin, M.; Burrell, A.; Imre, H.; Winter, J.; Lam, E.; Santtila, P. Linking serial sexual offences: Moving towards an ecologically valid test of the principles of crime linkage. *Leg. Criminol. Psychol.* **2019**, *24*, 123–140. [CrossRef]
37. Woodhams, J.; Labuschagne, G. A test of case linkage principles with solved and unsolved serial rapes. *J. Police Crim. Psychol.* **2012**, *27*, 85–98. [CrossRef]
38. Leclerc, B.; Wortley, R.; Dowling, C. Situational precipitators and interactive forces in sexual crime events involving adult offenders. *Crim. Justice Behav.* **2016**, *43*, 1600–1618. [CrossRef]
39. Chiu, Y.N.; Leclerc, B.; Reynald, D.M.; Wortley, R. Situational crime prevention in sexual offenses against women: Offenders tell us what works and what doesn't. *Int. J. Offender Ther. Comp. Criminol.* **2021**, *65*, 1055–1076. [CrossRef]
40. Rosenbaum, A.; Langhinrichsen-Rohling, J. Meta-research on violence and victims: The impact of data collection methods on findings and participants. *Violence Vict.* **2006**, *21*, 404–409. [CrossRef] [PubMed]
41. Muiruri, F. Dilemma as Post-Rape Care form is Rejected. Kenyan Woman. 2021. Available online: https://kw.awcfs.org/article/dilemma-as-post-rape-care-form-is-rejected/ (accessed on 31 July 2021).
42. Daly, K.; Bouhours, B. Rape and attrition in the legal process: A comparative analysis of five countries. *Crime Justice* **2010**, *39*, 565–650. [CrossRef]

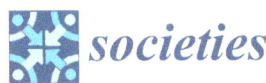

MDPI

Article

The Kenyan Survivors of Sexual Violence Network: Preserving Memory Evidence with a Bespoke Mobile Application to Increase Access to Vital Services and Justice

Laura M. Stevens [1], Elena Reid [1], Wangu Kanja [2], Sarah Rockowitz [1], Kari Davies [3], Shanaya Dosanjh [4], Brooke Findel [1] and Heather D. Flowe [1,*]

[1] School of Psychology, University of Birmingham, Birmingham B15 2TT, UK; lms825@student.bham.ac.uk (L.M.S.); reidellie1999@gmail.com (E.R.); SXR1005@student.bham.ac.uk (S.R.); BHF923@student.bham.ac.uk (B.F.)
[2] The Wangu Kanja Foundation, Nairobi P.O. Box 12608, Kenya; wangukanja@gmail.com
[3] School of Psychology, Bournemouth University, Dorset BH12 5BB, UK; kadavies@bournemouth.ac.uk
[4] School of Psychology, University of Warwick, Coventry CV4 7AL, UK; Shanaya.Dosanjh@warwick.ac.uk
* Correspondence: h.flowe@bham.ac.uk

Citation: Stevens, L.M.; Reid, E.; Kanja, W.; Rockowitz, S.; Davies, K.; Dosanjh, S.; Findel, B.; Flowe, H.D. The Kenyan Survivors of Sexual Violence Network: Preserving Memory Evidence with a Bespoke Mobile Application to Increase Access to Vital Services and Justice. *Societies* 2022, 12, 12. https://doi.org/10.3390/soc12010012

Academic Editors: Jaimee Mallion and Erika Gebo

Received: 6 December 2021
Accepted: 13 January 2022
Published: 19 January 2022

Publisher's Note: MDPI stays neutral with regard to jurisdictional claims in published maps and institutional affiliations.

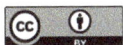
Abstract: Police interviews gather detailed information from witnesses about the perpetrator that is crucial for solving crimes. Research has established that interviewing witnesses immediately after the crime maintains memory accuracy over time. However, in some contexts, such as in conflict settings and low-income countries, witness interviews occur after long delays, which decreases survivors' access to vital services and justice. We investigated whether an immediate interview via a mobile phone application (SV_CaseStudy Mobile Application, hereafter MobApp) developed by the Kenyan Survivors of Sexual Violence Network preserves people's memory accuracy over time. Participants ($N = 90$) viewed a mock burglary and were then interviewed either immediately using MobApp or MobApp+ (which included additional questions about the offender's behaviour) and again one week later ($n = 60$), or solely after a one-week delay ($n = 30$). We found that memory accuracy one week later was higher for participants immediately interviewed with MobApp or MobApp+ compared to those interviewed solely after a one-week delay. Additionally, memory accuracy was maintained for those interviewed with the mobile application across the one-week period. These findings indicate that the mobile phone application is promising for preserving memory accuracy in contexts where crimes are reported to the police after a delay.

Keywords: gender-based violence; sexual violence; Kenya; memory; behavioural crime linkage; access to justice

1. Introduction

Statements and testimony given by witnesses, which include that of victim survivors and bystanders (e.g., the victim's family, community members), are vitally important in criminal investigations [1]. The information they provide often includes a description of the perpetrator's physical appearance and behaviours, which can aid in perpetrator identification and provide leads in securing and interpreting forensic evidence [2]. However, due to demands on police time and other resource constraints, there are often lengthy delays between the crime and when the police can gather statements from witnesses [3,4]. The length of the delay can affect a witness' ability to recollect, or recall, information about the crime. Research has found that recall is optimal immediately after a witnessed event; but, as the delay between the event and the first recall attempt increases, the number of correct details recalled decreases [5,6]. However, research has found that the sooner a witness is interviewed, the fewer details that they will forget about the crime over time [3]. This matters because a witness will provide statements several times over the course of justice proceedings, such as recalling the crime to first responders (e.g., human rights defenders, community health volunteers, police, medical personnel), criminal investigators, and jurors in court. Thus, a relatively early interview can preserve the witness' memory for longer, leading to more accurate memory evidence over time.

Interviewing witnesses soon after a crime, however, is challenging even in the best of circumstances (e.g., when a police station, well-trained interviewers, and a secure environment are available) [7]. Interviewing in sexual violence cases is especially difficult in conflict settings and contexts where insufficient resources are available for investigations and survivors are stigmatised, such as Kenya [8]. To overcome these obstacles, communities in Kenya are documenting sexual and gender-based violence (SGBV) incidents using a mobile application. This work is being organised by the Wangu Kanja Foundation (WKF), a Kenyan non-profit organisation that focuses on promoting prevention, protection, and response in ending sexual violence in the country. The vision of the foundation is towards a society that is safe and free from all forms of violence. The WKF convenes the Survivors of Sexual Violence in Kenya Network (hereafter the Network) that brings together survivors of sexual violence, which includes women, men, and children, to amplify their voices towards restoring their dignity and assisting survivors in accessing vital services and justice in a timely manner (e.g., police, medical, safe shelters, and other agencies that promote the safety of the victim).

The WKF has pioneered a mobile phone application (SV_CaseStudy Mobile Application, herein MobApp) to interview survivors, that allows survivors the opportunity to report and document anonymously should they wish to. Moreover, whilst anyone can utilise MobApp on their own or someone else's mobile device, currently MobApp is primarily being used by the Network, which spans across all 47 counties of Kenya. Members of the Network are sexual violence survivors who are also human rights defenders and community health volunteers, trained in a trauma sensitive manner to respond to incidents of SGBV within their community. The Network is using MobApp to interview survivors, following provision of informed consent, to obtain an early account of violations and track cases across the referral pathway (e.g., health, security, and justice mechanisms). MobApp records are currently held by the WKF; however, a survivor can access them at any point and share them with any involved parties. The WKF are hoping MobApp will be adopted in in the future in Kenya by other agencies along the case referral pathway.

This study tested the efficacy of MobApp in preserving memory over time, and explored whether adapting the app to include questions that enable serial crimes to be linked lead to more comprehensive accounts from witnesses. Behavioural crime linkage (BCL) uses the principles of behavioural consistency and distinctiveness to identify patterns of behaviour across a series of crimes, which can then be attributed to a serial offender. Research has shown that this type of behavioural analysis can be used to successfully link multiple crimes committed by the same offender [9]. Therefore, we studied whether incorporating questions about the offender's behaviour increases the amount of information gathered from witnesses about offences, and the offender's behaviour in particular, which in turn can be used to facilitate the application of BCL. This is particularly important in low-resource environments like Kenya, because BCL enables investigators to solve crimes more efficiently, and thus, could prevent future crimes from occurring. In what follows, we provide an overview of (1) the Kenyan context and work being done by communities with respect to documenting sexual offences; (2) research on techniques that help prevent memory loss over time; and (3) research on the use of BCL to link serial crimes. Thereafter, the aims and an overview of the current study are presented.

1.1. Kenyan Context

Nearly 41% of women in Kenya have experienced physical or sexual intimate partner violence in their lifetime and nearly 26% have experienced it in the last 12 months [10]. Gender inequality is rampant in Kenya, which ranks 135th out of 159 countries on the Gender Inequality Index, a measure that indexes inequality between women and men in reproductive health, empowerment, and labour market participation [11]. Further, sexual violence, which can be perpetrated against anyone, but most often is against women and girls, increases in Kenya in times of conflict, such as during postelection periods [12].

Poor data quality in Kenya makes sexual violence difficult to study. Researchers measure crime patterns using self-report surveys to gather information about incidents that, in many cases, happened long ago. Such data may not be accurate for a host of possible reasons, including forgetting, or respondents' fear of being judged, endangered, or penalised, which in turn leads to data incompleteness or inaccuracy [13]. As MobApp data is collected by human rights defenders, who are also trusted members of their communities, this potentially ameliorates some data validity concerns. For example, MobApp is widely distributed, and allows data to be gathered by survivors anonymously and relatively soon after the offence. Further, the data collected can be analysed in real time to identify emerging crime hotspots, which may prevent crime, as well as identify where vital services are needed.

1.2. Preventing Memory Failure

Best-practice interview techniques employ open-ended free recall prompts for eliciting statements from witnesses [14–16]. These prompts improve recall accuracy by allowing witnesses the opportunity to actively retrieve information from memory about the crime and freely report it using their own words. The WKF documents cases by prompting survivors to freely recall the crime. MobApp also includes specific questions about the perpetrator and the offence. Memory research suggests this may have a beneficial effect on survivors' ability to remember the crime over time during criminal investigations and judicial proceedings. This is vitally important in contexts where reporting to the authorities is often delayed (e.g., rural areas, times of conflict) and where the adjudication process is lengthy. In Kenya, crimes are seldom reported, and adjudications are rare, and as such, MobApp could turn the tide. Drawing on research about the vital role of an early interview in preserving memory [3], researchers recently found that allowing witnesses to write down their memories of a crime relatively soon afterwards preserves memory accuracy over time [3,17,18]. To our knowledge, there has been only one study investigating whether recalling a crime by recording it with a mobile application preserves memory. This app was developed by academic researchers in Australia, and they conducted an experimental investigation that found that research participants who used it to provide an initial account remembered more accurate information over time [19]. The present study sought to replicate and extend this previous research, working closely with the community Network.

1.3. MobApp and Behavioural Analysis

Kenya has a relatively low prosecution rate, particularly in cases of sexual violence, partly owing to resource constraints [20]. The use of a mobile application to gather information about an offender's behaviour could be a relatively low-cost, yet effective, method to gather intelligence about criminal perpetrators. This information could then be used to identify a behavioural pattern of offending across a series of offences based on an offender's *modus operandi* (MO), which allows for linking crimes committed by the same offender and more effectively identifying serial perpetrators. In the Global North, research has found that information about consistent and distinctive perpetrator behaviours established through the victim's description of the offence to the police can be used to link crimes committed by the same perpetrator [21,22]. More recent work indicates that these techniques are promising in the Global South in helping the police to solve serial offences [23,24]. While the use of BCL is the focus of this paper in terms of understanding how the information collected by witnesses could be used for the purposes of behavioural analysis, it is also worth noting that information about offending behaviour can also be used in other ways, such as implementing situational crime prevention strategies to protect communities [25], which uses offence data to identify high-risk circumstances and determine preventative measures that may limit crime opportunities [26]. Mobile applications have previously been piloted in Kenya to gather data for situational crime prevention purposes with some success [8]; for instance, Oduor et al. (2014) found good will among the population to using apps to report crimes anonymously. For the interested reader, Aransiola and Ceccato (2020) provide further information about the use of modern technology for situational crime prevention, the exploration of which is beyond the scope of this paper [27].

In the present study, we investigated whether asking witnesses questions about the perpetrator's behaviour increases the total amount and accuracy of information reported about the crime. Specifically, drawing on *spreading of activation* theory, we hypothesised that when witnesses are asked to recall behaviourally relevant details about the perpetrator, it will strengthen their memory not only for behaviourally relevant details, but also for other aspects of the crime. Spreading of activation theory states that memories exist in networks [28]. When one node of the network is activated, it triggers the activation of other related information in memory. This leads to a strengthening of related memories. Therefore, we predicted that witnesses who are asked for behaviourally relevant information would recall more information about the perpetrator's behaviour and the crime overall than their counterparts.

1.4. Overview of Present Study

The present study investigated whether an immediate recall attempt made via MobApp or MobApp+ preserves memory accuracy over a one-week period in comparison to a control group. We used a mock-crime experiment paradigm wherein participant witnesses watched a mock-crime video and then had their memory of the crime tested one week later. This approach is appropriate for our purposes because it allows for measuring memory accuracy. A field test using real crime reports would not allow us to test our predictions because the accuracy of the witnesses' accounts could not be established as ground truth would be unknown. Our design included two intervention conditions and a control condition to which our participants were randomly assigned. Participants in our intervention conditions provided an initial account of the crime using either MobApp alone, or MobApp+, which is an enhanced version of MobApp that has the same questions as MobApp plus ones about the offender's behaviour before, during, and after the offence. Participants in the intervention conditions returned one week later to give another recall account of the crime. Participants in the control condition did not provide an initial account using an app, but rather recalled the crime for the first time one week later. The control group parallels usual practice in Kenya and other countries around the world with regard to sexual offences, whereby survivors frequently provide a delayed account to the police [3,4]. Our participants were recruited from the University of Birmingham in the United Kingdom (UK), owing to the pandemic and the urgent need to collect data quickly to inform practice in the field. Elections are occurring next year in Kenya, and MobApp, if it is effective, will be an especially important tool, considering that sexual violence increases during these periods [12]. Further tests in the field with the Network are planned using the outcome of this trial.

2. Methods

2.1. Design

We employed a 3-interview condition (MobApp, MobApp+, no initial recall) x 2 time point (immediate, one week) mixed design, with interview condition as the between groups factor, and time point as a within-subjects factor for those in the MobApp and MobApp+ conditions. Participants were randomly assigned to one of three initial interview conditions (MobApp, MobApp+, no initial recall). Participants in the MobApp condition answered questions immediately after the crime that would normally be asked of users of MobApp in Kenya. Those in the MobApp+ condition answered the same questions, but they were also asked questions about the offender's behaviour before, during and after the crime. Those in the no initial recall condition did not have an interview immediately after the crime. All participants returned after a one-week delay and were asked to recall the mock crime.

The dependent variables included the total number of details recalled, recall accuracy rate, number of correct details recalled, number of incorrect details recalled, number of behaviourally relevant details (both correct and incorrect) recalled, recall accuracy rate of behaviourally relevant details, and confabulations (e.g., details not present or relevant to the mock-crime video), with the data conditioned on time point (immediate versus one-week later).

2.2. Participants

Participants (N = 90; M age = 21.84; SD = 5.46; age range 18–49 years; n = 64 female) were voluntarily recruited using University of Birmingham Sona Systems Research Participation Scheme (RPS, n = 66) and the online recruitment platform Prolific (n = 24). Participants were blind to their condition allocation (n = 30 participants per condition) and participants were either remunerated 2.5 course credits or £7.60 p/hr for their time. To be eligible to participate in the current study, participants had to be over the age of 17 and fluent in English. Ethics was obtained from the University of Birmingham's STEM Research Ethics Committee. All participants provided informed consent prior to study participation.

2.3. Procedure and Materials

Each participant completed the task independently, using the online survey platform Qualtrics. Participants were initially asked to provide demographic information regarding their age, gender, and ethnicity, before receiving written instructions that they were about to watch CCTV footage of a non-violent crime (the video was of a mock burglary). Participants were explicitly informed to pay careful attention to the video as they would be asked questions about it later. The video depicted a non-violent mock crime lasting 3 min and 43 s, where one man burglarised a house, taking household items (e.g., laptop and headphones) when no one was home. Burglary was considered an appropriate crime type to test our hypothesis, as it is less traumatic than sexual violence and many sexual violence crimes have been orchestrated in combination with burglaries [29]. The video was constructed to provide details relevant to BCL [30,31], as informed by Meenaghan et al. (2018) and Tonkin and Weeks (2021). To link crimes, analysts look for consistent and distinctive behaviours exhibited by the perpetrators when they select, enter, search, and exit a property. Thus, the video was constructed in a manner to provide details to recall in these areas (e.g., depicting the perpetrator carefully searching the property without destruction).

Following the video presentation, participants were provided instructions corresponding to their condition allocation. All participants initially completed a distractor task that asked them to count back in threes from 332 for 60 s.

2.3.1. Control Group

Following the distractor task, the control group were thanked for their participation and were reminded that there would be a follow-up session one week later.

2.3.2. MobApp

Within each recall survey, participants were instructed that they should provide an accurate account where possible, and to put "I don't know" if they were unsure to avoid guessing. Participants first completed a free recall text box, instructing them to recall what they saw in the video. No time or character limits were placed onto responses. They were then presented with questions from the WKF MobApp that has been adapted to be applicable for a burglary. Questions prompted the participant about any details they may not have remembered in the free recall. The seven questions asked participants what type of crime was portrayed in the video, what date and time of day they witnessed the event, where the event took place, if they knew the perpetrator, and how many perpetrators were involved.

2.3.3. MobApp+

The MobApp+ survey was the same as the MobApp survey but was extended to include behavioural items [30,31]. Like the MobApp condition, MobApp+ initially asked participants to freely recall what they could remember in a text box. Following the free recall responses, participants received 11 questions, asking them to describe the crime scene location, an estimate of the time of day of the incident, and whether any other witnesses were at the scene of the incident. The questions informed by BCL were split into three distinctive stages. The first stage included how the perpetrator selected and entered the target or property. These questions asked participants to describe the events in the order that they occurred, whether there was any evidence that the perpetrator was selecting a target or property, and how the perpetrator entered the property. The second stage referred to what occurred whilst the perpetrator was inside the property, committing the offence. Questions asked how the perpetrator located items they stole from the property, and how the perpetrator searched the property. The final stage of questions focused on how the crime scene was exited, whether there were any distinctive or memorable behaviours of the perpetrator, and if and how the perpetrator showed forensic awareness.

2.3.4. One-Week Recall

One week after their initial recall, participants were sent a follow-up survey link on Qualtrics. This survey asked them to freely recall what they could remember about the video they had previously witnessed into the text box provided. Participants completed their second recall task within 26 h of their original time slot. All participants were then thanked for their participation and debriefed, told the purpose of this study, and reminded they were able to withdraw their data within 72 h of participation.

2.4. Coding and Measures

Both time points (immediate, one week) were coded for the total number of correct and incorrect details as well as the total number of details recalled, recall accuracy rate (proportion of correct details recalled), number of confabulations, number of behaviourally relevant details recalled (correct and incorrect), and recall accuracy rate of behaviourally relevant details (proportion correct of the total number of behaviourally relevant details recalled).

Participants' recall was coded into details using a standardised template informed by prior research [32]. Recall was categorised into details pertaining to Action (A), Person (P), Object (O), or Setting (S). For example, in the mock-crime video, 'a white male leaving a property' was coded as: 'white (1-P) male (1-P) leaving (1-A) property (1-S)'. This would equate to four total details recalled. A sum of all details mentioned correct and incorrect formed a participant's total recall. Each detail was further coded for whether it was present within the mock-crime video (correct), was present within the mock-crime video and was not recalled correctly (incorrect), or was not present/relevant to the mock-crime video (confabulation).

What was considered a behaviourally relevant detail was informed by Meenaghan et al. (2018) and Tonkin and Weeks (2021), including behavioural details about how the perpetrator selected, entered, searched, and exited the property. A behaviourally relevant detail was defined as any information pertaining to an action the perpetrator committed or context to said action. For example, 'the man (1-P) rode off (1-A) on a bike (1-O)' was coded as three behaviourally relevant details. Subjective responses, such as 'house itself was worth a bit of money', were not coded.

2.5. Inter-Rater Reliability

To assess inter-rater reliability, 18 participant responses were randomly selected in each condition and coded independently by two researchers. Cohen's Kappa was computed for the measures displayed in Table 1. This analysis indicated acceptable levels of (moderate to high) inter-rater reliability for each variable. Discrepancies were resolved through discussion prior to analysis.

Table 1. Cohen's Kappa Assessing Inter-Rater Reliability.

	Total Details			Behaviourally Relevant	
	Correct	Incorrect	Confabulation	Correct	Incorrect
Cohen's kappa (κ)	0.90	0.91	1.00	0.90	0.86
p-value	<0.001	<0.001	<0.001	<0.001	<0.001

Table note: A *p*-value < 0.001 indicates that the level of inter-rater agreement observed is different from what would be achieved by chance alone.

3. Results

3.1. Recall at One Week

Table 2 displays results of one-way ANCOVAs that were conducted to compare each dependent variable across conditions at one-week recall, using word count at one-week recall as a covariate to control for output. An ANCOVA compares the means across the conditions to assess whether they are statistically different, whilst controlling for a variable that may confound results (e.g., total amount of output in words). A significant main effect of recall accuracy rate by condition was found, $F(2, 43) = 3.79$, $p = 0.040$, $\eta^2 p = 0.07$. Participants in the MobApp+ condition demonstrated the highest recall accuracy rate, followed by the MobApp condition and the control condition with a medium effect size (see Table 2 for descriptive statistics).

Table 2. Descriptive and Inferential Statistics for One-Way ANCOVAs.

		Condition			F	p
		MobApp+	MobApp	Control		
One-Week Recall	Total Recall	35.17 (3.70)	37.53 (4.35)	33.20 (4.35)	1.18	0.312
	Correct Recall	33.83 (3.49)	35.80 (4.16)	30.53 (3.92)	2.28	0.109
	Incorrect Recall	1.33 (0.46)	1.73 (0.46)	2.67 (0.61)	3.30	0.042 *
	Accuracy Rate	0.97 (0.01)	0.92 (0.03)	0.85 (0.05)	3.79	0.040 *
	Behaviourally Relevant Accuracy Rate	0.96 (0.01)	0.93 (0.03)	0.84 (0.05)	2.59	0.068

* *p* < 0.05.

Orthogonal comparisons were conducted to compare the two MobApp conditions (MobApp and MobApp+) against the control condition, and to compare the two MobApp conditions against one another. These planned comparisons revealed a significant difference in recall accuracy rate between both MobApp and MobApp+ combined in comparison to the control group, $F(1, 87) = 5.32$, $p = 0.023$, $\eta^2 p = 0.06$. There was no significant difference in recall accuracy rate between MobApp and MobApp+ ($p = 0.170$). Therefore, participants given an initial interview had an increased recall accuracy rate in comparison to no initial recall at one-week final test (see Table 2).

A significant main effect of total number of incorrect details recalled by condition was obtained, $F(2, 86) = 3.30$, $p = 0.042$, $\eta^2 p = 0.07$, a medium effect size for condition (see Table 2 for descriptive statistics). Planned comparisons indicated a significant difference in the number of incorrect details recalled in the MobApp conditions combined in comparison to the control condition, $F(1, 87) = 6.65$, $p = 0.012$, $\eta^2 p = 0.07$. There was no significant difference in the number of incorrect details recalled between MobApp+ and MobApp ($p = 0.784$). Therefore, an initial recall attempt reduced the number of incorrect details recalled at one-week final test. For all other inferential statistics and descriptive statistics refer to Table 2.

3.2. MobApp Conditions Compared: Recall over Time

Additional analyses examined whether being questioned about the behaviour of the offender within the phone application increased the recall accuracy rate of reporting or the number of correct details recalled one week later. We conducted mixed ANCOVAs (2 time point × 2 MobApp interview conditions) for all dependent variables, with word count for each time point entered as covariates; results are displayed in Table 3. A mixed ANCOVA compares whether the means differ between conditions and/or across the two time points, as well as whether the use of MobApp differentially affects recall performance depending on delay.

Table 3. Descriptive and Inferential Statistics for Repeated-Measures ANCOVAs on each of the Dependent Variables.

	MobApp	MobApp+	Condition	Time	Condition × Time
Total Recall					
Immediate Recall	47.93 (4.51)	78.10 (6.46)	$F(1,56) = 0.68$ ns	$F(1,56) = 9.76$ **	$F(1,56) = 0.00$ ns
One-Week Recall	37.53 (4.35)	35.17 (3.70)			
Correct					
Immediate Recall	45.90 (4.35)	75.73 (6.27)	$F(1,56) = 0.13$ ns	$F(1,56) = 8.32$ **	$F(1,56) = 1.41$ ns
One-Week Recall	35.80 (4.16)	33.83 (3.49)			
Incorrect					
Immediate Recall	2.03 (0.49)	2.37 (0.45)	$F(1,56) = 1.19$ ns	$F(1,56) = 4.26$ *	$F(1,56) = 2.58$ ns
One-Week Recall	1.73 (0.46)	1.33 (0.46)			
Accuracy Rate					
Immediate Recall	0.96 (0.01)	0.97 (0.01)	$F(1,56) = 2.45$ ns	$F(1,56) = 1.13$ ns	$F(1,56) = 0.36$ ns
One-Week Recall	0.92 (0.03)	0.97 (0.01)			
Behaviourally Relevant Accuracy Rate					
Immediate Recall	0.96 (0.01)	0.97 (0.01)	$F(1,56) = 1.78$ ns	$F(1,56) = 2.04$ ns	$F(1,56) = 0.13$ ns
One-Week Recall	0.93 (0.03)	0.96 (0.01)			

* $p < 0.05$. ** $p < 0.01$.

Significant main effects of time were found for total details recalled ($F(1, 56) = 9.76$, $p = 0.003$, $\eta^2 p = 0.15$), total correct details recalled ($F(1, 56) = 8.32$, $p = 0.006$, $\eta^2 p = 0.13$), and total incorrect details recalled ($F(1, 56) = 4.26$, $p = 0.044$, $\eta^2 p = 0.07$), with mean recall decreasing over time. Thus, both the number of correct and incorrect details recalled decreased as a function of time. No significant main effects of time were found for the recall accuracy rate, or for the recall accuracy rate of behaviourally relevant details. No significant main effects of condition or interaction effects were found for any of the dependent variables. Therefore, the two versions of MobApp were comparable regarding recall across time points.

4. Discussion

We tested whether MobApp, a mobile application pioneered by a community Network in Kenya to document crimes, slows the rate of forgetting. We found that a recall attempt given immediately after witnessing a mock crime using MobApp or MobApp+ preserved the memory recall accuracy rate over a one-week period and led to increased recall accuracy in comparison to a control group. These findings are vitally important, as they indicate that MobApp can preserve memory recall over time. Memory preservation can improve the ability of survivors in communities with low resources to access justice. This is the first study to evaluate the efficacy of MobApp as a tool that preserves memory over time and that elicits information about the suspect's behaviour for BCL purposes. Next, we will discuss these findings in turn.

4.1. Memory Preservation over Time

Regardless of whether MobApp included prompts for the survivor to report information about the perpetrator's behaviour, the recall accuracy rate did not decrease over time. Recall accuracy was high immediately after the crime and one week later for those who used MobApp to give an immediate initial account. This finding is in line with previous research findings that an early initial recall attempt preserves memory accuracy across time [3,19]. Ours was the first study to extend these findings to the Kenyan community initiative MobApp. Previous research has found that participants are frequently accurate when they can freely recall details [33]. We found that an initial recall attempt using the community driven MobApp or the modified MobApp+ preserved recall accuracy rates across time, which means in practice that the community can use MobApp to gather accurate and essential details that can further investigations and prosecutions.

While the rate at which participants were accurate did not decrease over time for those who used the mobile application, the total number of details recalled did decrease over time. Specifically, participants in the MobApp condition and the behaviourally enhanced MobApp+ condition recalled more details in total (both correct and incorrect) in their initial recall attempt compared to one week later. These results do not replicate what is typically found in research on the benefit of an early initial recall attempt [3,34]. Previous research has found that participants who gave an early initial recall account maintain a similar number of total details recalled at initial test and final test [3,34]. The current research may not have replicated these findings for several reasons. First, over the one-week delay period, participants may have become increasingly stringent about the memories they reported, which in turn served to decrease the amount of information they reported, and this helped them maintain accuracy over time [33]. Put differently, witnesses may apply a strict reporting criterion, which preserves accuracy, but this comes at the expense of the completeness of the account [35]. Alternatively, the initial recall test prompted participants to freely recall the crime, and then prompted participants to recall information about the perpetrator's behaviour. In contrast, the final recall test included only a free recall prompt. This may have suggested to participants to report the same information as they had reported on the initial free recall account, leading them to leave out behavioural details on the final test that they would have reported had they been prompted for it.

Finally, this research had to be conducted using online survey platforms owing to the pandemic-related UK stay at home orders. This limited our ability to establish rapport with our participants, which is important in making people feel comfortable and motivated to disclose information [36]. On the ground in Kenya, a member of the Network collects the survivor's testimony in person using MobApp. As a result of this they can establish rapport with the survivor, which may lead to a greater number of details being disclosed than if the data were collected online.

We found that MobApp and MobApp+ led to a higher rate of recall accuracy one week later in comparison to the control group, which did not have an initial recall attempt. The control group represents the situation in most countries, wherein survivors of violence often delay their reporting to the police. Our work shows an initial recall attempt using a mobile application immediately after the crime can preserve accuracy, which is vital if survivors elect to report to the police after a delay. Participants in the MobApp+ condition did have the highest accuracy rates on average, albeit this difference was not statistically significant. Thus, we tentatively conclude that MobApp+ may potentially lead to the highest rate of accuracy over other known approaches when used by community actors documenting incidents of violence.

4.2. Behaviorally Relevant Details

The use of the mobile applications also led to increased recall accuracy for behaviourally relevant details compared to the control condition, although the difference was not statistically significant. Given these results, we would encourage community organisations to prompt survivors for behaviourally relevant details. First, doing so does not decrease accuracy. Second, behaviourally relevant details can be used to link crimes together, helping to provide evidence and aid investigations to bring serial offenders to apprehension, thus preventing further offences [21–24]. Additionally, and as noted above, behaviourally relevant details can also be important for other types of analyses, such as indicating geographical and temporal crime patterns to inform situational crime prevention strategies. In contexts such as Kenya, where there are limited resources, this information may be strategically important for developing preventative measures, such as increased police or community surveillance at certain times or in certain locations [37].

4.3. Limitations and Future Directions

We need to learn more about the experiences of communities who are using mobile applications to document crimes and in wide ranging contexts. The present study was necessarily limited to an experimental paradigm that tested people's ability to remember a mock crime over a one-week period. In real world cases there are often delays of months or years in between reporting [3,4]. Further, the witnesses' duration of exposure to the culprit in real world crimes, including rape, is relatively long compared to the exposure time used in the present study [38]. Delay and duration of exposure can affect how strong the witness' memory is of the crime. However, there is no theoretical reason to expect that remembering would be better in the control compared to the MobApp conditions depending on memory strength. Further, under conditions where memory is initially exceptionally weak, or exceptionally strong, using an app would have less of an effect on preserving memory over time.

MobApp is used predominantly in Kenya to document cases of SGBV. However, for ethical reasons, the mock crime we used was not an incident of SGBV. There has been debate about the impact of traumatic events (e.g., SGBV) on memory, with some researchers concluding that incidents of trauma are remembered less vividly than other types of events [39], while others maintain that traumatic events are remembered in greater detail than other events [40]. Nevertheless, all other things being equal, we know of no theoretical reason why trauma would diminish the benefits of an early interview in preserving memory.

Additionally, whilst the current study did not investigate memory for SGBV within a Kenyan sample, the results likely generalise to Kenyans. The effect of an initial recall attempt has been found in several countries (e.g., Spain, Mexico, the Netherlands, Australia) [41]. Therefore, there is good reason to expect that the findings generalise to people in Kenya. Finally, in Kenya, MobApp provides an opportunity to amplify survivors' voices. Survivors are often silenced by the culture of stigma and shame surrounding SGBV in Kenya [42], and this frequently leads to survivors not reporting these crimes to the police. For survivors who do decide to report, the quality of their statements given to the police may be compromised because the police have insufficient resources to support the training of officers to conduct interviews using evidence-based practice [8]. In Kenya, the forms used to record the crime include little space to record the survivor's account. Further, a culture of impunity that silences many victims currently reigns in Kenya [43]. Thus, an ongoing issue is the need to enable survivors to report in an effective manner the crimes that occur against them. The Network members are trusted within their communities, and this leads to increased disclosure [44,45]. Therefore, providing Network members with a tool that documents cases and preserves recall accuracy over time is a positive development.

The use of human rights defenders to document incidents of SGBV in Kenya helps to overcome some of the obstacles that preclude survivors from accessing a mobile application. In Kenya, currently 18% of the population are illiterate [46]; thus, it is crucial in many cases that a Network member is available to aid in the documentation the case. MobApp currently does not handle voice recordings, and even if it did, this would require additional data usage, which would be expensive and cost prohibitive for many people in Kenya. Whilst almost everyone in Kenya owns a mobile device, only an estimated 40% have access to the Internet [47]. Therefore, arming human rights defenders with mobile devices to document the survivor's account is essential. Our current research is evaluating methods to train communities using MobApp to document cases using best-practice interview techniques. This is critical because community organisations are often the first responders and the ones to obtain the survivor's account. The quality of an initial account plays a crucial role in case progression and criminal justice proceedings [48,49]. If the account is taken using best practice, this can increase the likelihood of a successful prosecution. This research is vital because research has found that it is difficult to conduct an interview, even when interviewers have specialist training [50]. In view of this, our current co-developed research agenda seeks to build the capacity of the WKF to document cases through sustainable training packages that are freely available and instil best-practice interview techniques using a survivor-centred approach that seeks to minimise re-traumatisation during the process.

Finally, the use of mobile applications by communities to document crimes is likely to rise, particularly in the times of COVID-19, wherein police stations can be even harder to reach owing to lockdowns and curfews [44]. Thus, research on the impact of such apps on memory accuracy is critical. There is evidence to suggest that communities are receptive to using apps like MobApp. In Kenya, Oduor et al. (2014) examined the use of mobile applications as a tool for situational crime prevention. The mobile application they investigated allows users to receive crime updates, report crimes, search for lost friends, contact the police, and locate crime hotspots. Mobile applications of this kind may be particularly important in contexts like Kenya, wherein survivors may be reluctant to report sexual offences to the police owing to fear and stigma, or because they cannot travel to a police station. In Oduor et al. (2014), participants reported that they would likely use an app to report crime, as it enables reporting of the incident anonymously without the need to go to the police station. Given this context, MobApp may prove to be especially valuable.

5. Conclusions

We found that MobApp can preserve recall accuracy over a one-week period. This community-developed tool is also effective in the documentation of information about the perpetrator's behaviour, which can be vital in linking serial crimes. Our results are promising for low-resource contexts like Kenya, where communities are seeking to document crimes to illustrate and understand the nature of the violations that are occurring. Our research indicates that MobApp preserves memory accuracy over time, which is vital considering that crimes are infrequently reported, and that among those that are reported, there is often a long delay between the crime and adjudication

Author Contributions: Conceptualization, L.M.S., H.D.F., W.K. and K.D.; methodology, L.M.S., H.D.F., E.R. and K.D.; formal analysis, L.M.S., E.R. and H.D.F.; resources, W.K.; data curation, E.R., S.D., L.M.S. and B.F.; writing—original draft preparation, L.M.S., S.R., K.D. and H.D.F.; writing—review and editing, L.M.S., S.R., S.D., K.D., B.F., E.R. and H.D.F.; supervision, H.D.F.; project administration, S.R.; funding acquisition, H.D.F. and W.K. All authors have read and agreed to the published version of the manuscript.

Funding: This research was funded by AHRC Grant AH/T008091/1 (to HDF and the Wangu Kanja Foundation).

Institutional Review Board Statement: This study was conducted according to guidelines of the British Psychological Society and approved by University of Birmingham's STEM Research Ethics Committee (ERN_18-0031AP8, date of approval 22 February 2021).

Informed Consent Statement: Informed consent was obtained from all subjects involved in the study.

Data Availability Statement: Data can be found here: https://osf.io/47ct8/?view_only=08c633da9 79b4dfa961ad488817c97cc (accessed on 13 January 2022).

Acknowledgments: We are grateful to the Wangu Kanja Foundation and the Survivors of Sexual Violence Network Kenya for providing access to SV_CaseStudy Mobile Application.

Conflicts of Interest: The authors declare no conflict of interest. The funders had no role in the design of the study; in the collection, analyses, or interpretation of data; in the writing of the manuscript, or in the decision to publish the results.

References

1. Hope, L.; Gabbert, F.; Fisher, R.P.; Jamieson, K. Protecting and enhancing eyewitness memory: The impact of an initial recall attempt on performance in an investigative interview. *Appl. Cogn. Psychol.* **2014**, *28*, 304–313. [CrossRef]
2. Satin, G.E.; Fisher, R.P. Investigative utility of the Cognitive Interview: Describing and finding perpetrators. *Law Hum. Behav.* **2019**, *43*, 491–506. [CrossRef] [PubMed]
3. Gabbert, F.; Hope, L.; Fisher, R.P. Protecting eyewitness evidence: Examining the efficacy of a self-administered interview tool. *Law Hum. Behav.* **2009**, *33*, 298–307. [CrossRef] [PubMed]
4. Read, J.D.; Connolly, D.A. The effects of delay on long-term memory for witnessed events. In *The Handbook of Eyewitness Psychology. Memory for Events*; Toglia, M.P., Read, J.D., Ross, D.F., Lindsay, R.C.L., Eds.; Lawrence Erlbaum Associates Publishers: Mahwah, NJ, USA, 2007; Volume 1, pp. 117–155.
5. Wixted, J.T.; Ebbesen, E.B. On the form of forgetting. *Psychol. Sci.* **1991**, *2*, 409–415. [CrossRef]
6. Wixted, J.T.; Ebbesen, E.B. Genuine power curves in forgetting: A quantitative analysis of individual subject forgetting functions. *Mem. Cogn.* **1997**, *25*, 731–739. [CrossRef]
7. Wright, R.; Powell, M.B. Investigative interviewers' perceptions of their difficulty in adhering to open-ended questions with child witnesses. *Int. J. Police Sci. Manag.* **2006**, *8*, 316–325. [CrossRef]
8. Oduor, C.; Acosta, F.; Makhanu, E. The adoption of mobile technology as a tool for situational crime prevention in Kenya. In Proceedings of the 2014 IST-Africa Conference Proceedings (IEEE), Pointe aux Piments, Mauritius, 7–9 May 2014.
9. Woodhams, J.; Hollin, C.R.; Bull, R. The psychology of linking crimes: A review of the evidence. *Leg. Criminol. Psychol.* **2007**, *12*, 233–249. [CrossRef]
10. Kenya National Bureau of Statistics. *Kenya Demographic and Health Survey 2014*; The DHS Program, ICF International: Rockville, MD, USA, 2015.
11. United Nations Development Programme. *Human Development Report 2016*; United Nations Development Programme: New York, NY, USA, 2016.
12. Human Rights Watch. *"I Just Sit and Wait to Die" Reparations for Survivors of Kenya's 2007–2008 Post-Election Sexual Violence*; Human Rights Watch: New York, NY, USA, 2016.
13. Cullen, C. Method matters: Underreporting of intimate partner violence in Nigeria and Rwanda. *World Bank Policy Res. Work. Pap.* **2020**, *9274*, 1–43.
14. Lamb, M.E.; Brown, D.A.; Hershkowitz, I.; Orbach, Y.; Esplin, P.W. *Tell Me what Happened: Questioning Children about Abuse*; John Wiley & Sons: Hoboken, NJ, USA, 2018.
15. Lamb, M.E.; Hershkowitz, I.; Orbach, Y.; Esplin, P.W. *Tell Me what Happened: Structured Investigative Interviews of Child Victims and Witnesses*; John Wiley & Sons: Hoboken, NJ, USA, 2011; Volume 56.
16. Paulo, R.M.; Albuquerque, P.B.; Saraiva, M.; Bull, R. The enhanced cognitive interview: Testing appropriateness perception, memory capacity and error estimate relation with report quality. *Appl. Cogn. Psychol.* **2015**, *29*, 536–543. [CrossRef]
17. Gabbert, F.; Hope, L.; Fisher, R.P.; Jamieson, K. Protecting against misleading post-event information with a self-administered interview. *Appl. Cogn. Psychol.* **2012**, *26*, 568–575. [CrossRef]
18. Hope, L.; Gabbert, F.; Fisher, R.P. From laboratory to the street: Capturing witness memory using the Self-Administered Interview. *Leg. Criminol. Psychol.* **2011**, *16*, 211–226. [CrossRef]
19. Paterson, H.; Chevroulet, C.; van Golde, C.; Cowdery, N.; Kemp, R. Protecting eyewitness memory using a smartphone app. *Psychiatry Psychol. Law* **2021**, 1–18, *(manuscript under review)*. [CrossRef]
20. OSAC. Kenya 2020 Crime & Safety Report. 2020. Available online: https://www.osac.gov/Country/Kenya/Content/Detail/Report/50c57c03-c161-4f9c-8942-182082896065 (accessed on 14 January 2022).
21. Bennell, C.; Bloomfield, S.; Snook, B.; Taylor, P.; Barnes, C. Linkage analysis in cases of serial burglary: Comparing the performance of university students, police professionals, and a logistic regression model. *Psychol. Crime Law* **2010**, *16*, 507–524. [CrossRef]
22. Bennell, C.; Jones, N.J.; Melnyk, T. Addressing problems with traditional crime linking methods using receiver operating characteristic analysis. *Leg. Criminol. Psychol.* **2009**, *14*, 293–310. [CrossRef]
23. Woodhams, J.; Bennell, C. *Crime Linkage: Theory, Research, and Practice*; CRC Press: Boca Raton, FL, USA, 2014.
24. Woodhams, J.; Labuschagne, G. South African serial rapists: The offenders, their victims, and their offenses. *Sex. Abus.* **2012**, *24*, 544–574. [CrossRef] [PubMed]
25. Chiu, Y.N.; Leclerc, B.; Reynald, D.M.; Wortley, R. Situational crime prevention in sexual offenses against women: Offenders tell us what works and what doesn't. *Int. J. Offender Ther. Comp. Criminol.* **2021**, *65*, 1055–1076. [CrossRef]
26. Leclerc, B.; Chiu, Y.N.; Cale, J.; Cook, A. Sexual violence against women through the lens of environmental criminology: Toward the accumulation of evidence-based knowledge and crime prevention. *Eur. J. Crim. Policy Res.* **2016**, *22*, 593–617. [CrossRef]
27. Aransiola, T.J.; Ceccato, V. The role of modern technology in rural situational crime prevention: A review of the literature. In *Rural Crime Prevention: Theory, Tactics and Techniques*, 1st ed.; Harkness, A., Ed.; Routledge: London, UK, 2020; pp. 58–72.
28. Anderson, J.R. A spreading activation theory of memory. *J. Verbal Learn. Verbal Behav.* **1983**, *22*, 261–295. [CrossRef]

29. Pedneault, A.; Beauregard, E.; Harris, D.A.; Knight, R.A. Rationally irrational: The case of sexual burglary. *Sex. Abus.* **2015**, *27*, 376–397. [CrossRef]
30. Meenaghan, A.; Nee, C.; Van Gelder, J.L.; Otte, M.; Vernham, Z. Getting closer to the action: Using the virtual enactment method to understand burglary. *Deviant Behav.* **2018**, *39*, 437–460. [CrossRef]
31. Tonkin, M.; Weeks, M.J. Crime linkage practice in New Zealand. *J. Criminol. Res. Policy Pract.* **2021**, *7*, 63–76. [CrossRef]
32. Wright, A.M.; Holliday, R.E. Enhancing the recall of young, young–old and old–old adults with cognitive interviews. *Appl. Cogn. Psychol.* **2007**, *21*, 19–43. [CrossRef]
33. Goldsmith, M.; Koriat, A.; Pansky, A. Strategic regulation of grain size in memory reporting over time. *J. Mem. Lang.* **2005**, *52*, 505–525. [CrossRef]
34. Ebbesen, E.B.; Rienick, C.B. Retention interval and eyewitness memory for events and personal identifying attributes. *J. Appl. Psychol.* **1998**, *83*, 745–762. [CrossRef] [PubMed]
35. Weber, N.; Brewer, N. Eyewitness recall: Regulation of grain size and the role of confidence. *J. Exp. Psychol. Appl.* **2008**, *14*, 50–60. [CrossRef]
36. Lamb, M.E.; Orbach, Y.; Hershkowitz, I.; Esplin, P.W.; Horowitz, D. A structured forensic interview protocol improves the quality and informativeness of investigative interviews with children: A review of research using the NICHD Investigative Interview Protocol. *Child Abus. Negl.* **2007**, *31*, 1201–1231. [CrossRef]
37. Farrington, D.P.; Welsh, B.C. *Effects of Improved Street Lighting on Crime: A Systematic Review*; Home Office: London, UK, 2002.
38. Flowe, H.D.; Carline, A.; Karoğlu, N. Testing the reflection assumption: A comparison of eyewitness ecology in the laboratory and criminal cases. *Int. J. Evid. Proof* **2018**, *22*, 239–261. [CrossRef]
39. Koss, M.P.; Figueredo, A.J.; Bell, I.; Tharan, M.; Tromp, S. Traumatic memory characteristics: A cross-validated mediational model of response to rape among employed women. *J. Abnorm. Psychol.* **1996**, *105*, 421–432. [CrossRef]
40. Porter, S.; Birt, A.R. Is traumatic memory special? A comparison of traumatic memory characteristics with memory for other emotional life experiences. *Appl. Cogn. Psychol. Off. J. Soc. Appl. Res. Mem. Cogn.* **2001**, *15*, S101–S117. [CrossRef]
41. Horry, R.; Hughes, C.; Sharma, A.; Gabbert, F.; Hope, L. A meta-analytic review of the Self-Administered Interview©: Quantity and accuracy of details reported on initial and subsequent retrieval attempts. *Appl. Cogn. Psychol.* **2021**, *35*, 428–444. [CrossRef]
42. Owiti, J.A.; Otieno, P.E.; Kanja, W. *Survivors of Sexual Violence Consultative Forum Report*; Wanju Kanja Foundation: Nairobi, Kenya, 2018.
43. National Crime Research Centre. *Gender Based Violence in Kenya*; National Crime Research Centre: Nairobi, Kenya, 2014.
44. Flowe, H.D.; Rockowitz, S.; Rockey, J.; Kanja, W.; Kamau, C.; Colloff, M.; Kauldar, J.; Woodhams, J.; Davies, K. *Sexual and Other Forms of Violence During the COVID-19 Pandemic Emergency in Kenyas*; University of Birmingham Institute for Global Innovation: Birmingham, UK, 2020.
45. Rockowitz, S.; Stevens, L.M.; Rockey, J.C.; Smith, L.L.; Ritchie, J.; Colloff, M.F.; Kanja, W.; Cotton, J.; Njoroge, D.; Kamau, C.; et al. Patterns of sexual violence against adults and children during the COVID-19 pandemic in Kenya: A prospective cross-sectional study. *BMJ Open* **2021**, *11*, e048636. [CrossRef] [PubMed]
46. World Bank. Available online: https://data.worldbank.org/indicator/SE.ADT.LITR.ZS?locations=KE (accessed on 8 January 2022).
47. Connecting Africa. Available online: http://www.connectingafrica.com/author.asp?section_id=761&doc_id=768744 (accessed on 8 January 2022).
48. Campbell, R.; Adams, A.E.; Wasco, S.M.; Ahrens, C.E.; Sefl, T. Training interviewers for research on sexual violence: A qualitative study of rape survivors' recommendations for interview practice. *Violence Against Women* **2009**, *15*, 595–617. [CrossRef] [PubMed]
49. Elmir, R.; Schmied, V.; Jackson, D.; Wilkes, L. Interviewing people about potentially sensitive topics. *Nurse Res.* **2011**, *19*, 12–16. [CrossRef]
50. Powell, M.B. Designing effective training programs for investigative interviewers of children. *Curr. Issues Crim. Justice* **2008**, *20*, 189–208. [CrossRef]

MDPI

St. Alban-Anlage 66

4052 Basel

Switzerland

Tel. +41 61 683 77 34

Fax +41 61 302 89 18

www.mdpi.com

Societies Editorial Office

E-mail: societies@mdpi.com

www.mdpi.com/journal/societies

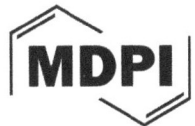